High-Yield Pharmacology

Second Edition

High-Yield Pharmacology

Second Edition

Daryl Christ, PhD
Associate Professor of Pharmacology
South Bend Center for Medical Education
Indiana University School of Medicine
Notre Dame, Indiana

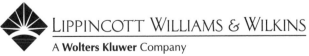
LIPPINCOTT WILLIAMS & WILKINS
A **Wolters Kluwer** Company
Philadelphia · Baltimore · New York · London
Buenos Aires · Hong Kong · Sydney · Tokyo

Editor: Neil Marquardt
Managing Editor: Daniel Pepper
Marketing Manager: Scott Lavine
Production Editor: Jennifer Ajello
Designer: Risa Clow
Compositor: Peirce Graphics
Printer: Data Reproduction Corporation

Library of Congress Cataloging-in-Publication Data

Christ, Daryl.
    High-yield pharmacology / Daryl Christ.—2nd ed.
        p. ; cm.
    Includes index.
    ISBN 0-7817-4512-8
    1. Pharmacology—Outlines, syllabi, etc.   I.   Title.
    [DNLM: 1. Pharmacology–Outlines.   QV 18.2 C554h 2003]
    RM301.14.C48   2003
    615′.1—dc21

                                                                2003042344

Preface

First, the name is pronounced Chrĭst, as in Christ-ian, Christ-mas, or Christ-opher. As the son of farmers, Esther and George Christ, I learned at an early age to reduce life to a few simple principles. In my 30 years of teaching pharmacology, the benefits of using such an approach to prepare students for the United States Medical Licensing Examination (USMLE) have become obvious.

The underlying premise for the *High Yield Pharmacology* book is that **a good grasp of the major concepts of pharmacology is better than a poor grasp of all the concepts of pharmacology.** In this regard, **it is best to study the drugs as classes**, rather than as individual drugs. **Begin by studying the prototype drug for each class, and then expand on this by studying how the other drugs in the class differ from the prototype. Only generic names are used on the examination.** However, in this book the trade name, or an example of one trade name for that generic drug, has been provided for informational purposes. These trade names are indicated in parentheses and italic type and are placed directly after the corresponding generic name. No dosages and **very few chemical structures need to be remembered** for the USMLE Step 1. **Memorization of long lists of mundane side effects, detailed kinetic properties, and detailed mechanisms of action is usually not required. Instead, the most important or the unique properties of the drugs should be studied. Many pharmacological principles evolved from the autonomic drugs, so a thorough understanding of this class of drugs is essential.**

For those desiring quick reviews, two approaches can be used. The bold printed text can be studied. Alternatively, studying the index will help you remember the class for each drug.

High Yield Pharmacology is based on a review guide that I first wrote in 1988 called *Pharmacology in a Nutshell*. This has been adopted by each statewide Indiana University medical class, and in recent years the classes have taken over the task of copying, binding, and distributing the *Pharmacology in a Nutshell* to all the Indiana University sophomore medical students. The students have frequently commented that most of the material needed for the USMLE, Step 1 was covered in *Pharmacology in a Nutshell*. Since 1991, I have also been presenting a 7-hour review of pharmacology, given in 1 day, to each statewide Indiana University sophomore medical class before the USMLE Step 1.

My background in teaching medical pharmacology began at the University of Arkansas College of Medicine in 1970. I left Arkansas in 1983 to take a position on the faculty of the Indiana University School of Medicine at the South Bend Center for Medical Education, where I still teach. During that time, I have received a Pre-Clinical Science Golden Apple Award (1981), a Runner-Up Pre-Clinical Science Golden Apple Award (1983), Outstanding Professor in Basic Sciences Teaching Awards (1993, 2002) and a Teaching Excellence Recognition Award (1998).

The statewide program at Indiana University is a truly unique medical education program, in which half of each freshman and sophomore medical class attends at Indianapolis and the other half of the class is divided among 8 university campuses for their basic science courses. The small Center for Medical Education at South Bend provides me with an opportunity to teach the complete pharmacology course by myself to a group of 14–16 sophomore medical students. This format allows for consistent coverage of all the material in an organized fashion.

This review book, *High Yield Pharmacology*, in a format proven to be effective for medical students studying for USMLE Step 1, similarly provides consistent, concise, and comprehensive coverage.

Daryl Christ

Acknowledgments

The author would like to acknowledge some of the people who have had a major impact on his life. First and foremost are his wife Bonnie and his son Alan, who, as an artist and an architect, respectively, always remind him that life is more than just science. The author would also like to acknowledge his parents, Esther and George Christ, and older brothers, Don and Duane Christ, who were so important during his formative and later years. Others will recognize their initials, including friends from Lakota High School in Iowa (DWC), Wartburg College (DAH and CDK), University of Iowa (JRS), and Loyola University in Chicago (JWG, TJS, JPG, PSG, RSJ, and NJD).

It has also been the author's good fortune to work with some excellent pharmacologists and educators, including Leslie C. Blaber, Alexander G. Karczmar, and Syogoro Nishi at Loyola University in Chicago; Werner E. Flacke and Donald E. McMillan at the University of Arkansas; Henry R. Besch, Jr., Thomas A. Troeger, and John F. O'Malley at Indiana University; and Howard J. Saz at the University of Notre Dame.

Contents

1
General Principles

I. ABSORPTION AND DISTRIBUTION OF DRUGS

A. **Pharmacokinetics** is the study of the movement of drugs into and out of the body, including **uptake, distribution, biotransformation,** and **elimination.**

B. The movement of drugs across cell membranes usually occurs by **diffusion.**

C. The rate of diffusion is high if:

1. **The unionized form of a drug has a high lipid solubility.**
  a. The lipid solubility is related to the oil-water partition coefficient.
  b. Cell membranes are basically lipoidal in nature, and only lipid soluble substances will diffuse through them.

2. **A large proportion of the drug is present in the unionized form.**
  a. **Only the unionized form can cross cell membranes,** because the ionized form will have a very low solubility in lipids.
  b. The equilibrium between the ionized (A^-) and unionized (HA) forms of a weak acid is:

$$HA \rightleftharpoons H^+ + A^-$$

  c. The proportion of unionized drug will depend on the pH and can be determined with the Henderson-Hasselbalch equation.
  d. For a drug that is a weak acid, the equation is:

$$pK_a = pH + \log\frac{[\text{unionized}]}{[\text{ionized}]}$$

  e. Weak bases also dissociate, and the equilibrium for a weak base is:

$$B + H^+ \rightleftharpoons BH^+$$

  f. The Henderson-Hasselbalch relationship for a weak base is:

$$pK_a = pH + \log\frac{[\text{ionized}]}{[\text{unionized}]}$$

  g. The ratio of unionized to ionized drug concentrations for a weak base at a given pH is the inverse of the ratio for a weak acid.

  h. When the pH equals the pK_a, 50% of a drug will be ionized and 50% will be unionized.

    i. The biggest changes in the amounts of ionized and unionized drug occur with pH changes near the pK_a.

  3. **The membrane is thin.**

  4. **The membrane is porous.** Porosity is especially important for water-soluble drugs.

  5. **The surface area of the membrane is large.**

  6. **The difference in concentrations on the two sides of the membrane is large.**

  7. **The diffusion constant, based on molecular size, molecular shape, and temperature, is large.**

D. At the **low pH** in the stomach:

  1. **Weak acids are well absorbed** because most of the drug is unionized.

  2. **Weak bases are poorly absorbed** because most of the drug is ionized.

E. **Ion trapping** occurs with weak acids and weak bases if there is a difference in pH on the two sides of a membrane.

  1. **The ionized form of the drug will be trapped on one side.**

    a. The ionized form of a **weak base** will be trapped on the side with the **lower pH.**

    b. The ionized form of a **weak acid** will be trapped on the side with the **higher pH.**

  2. Figure 1–1 illustrates ion trapping for a weak acid with a pK_a of 6.4. At equilibrium, the unionized concentrations on either side of the membrane will be equal, but 91% of the drug will be in the compartment at pH 7.4.

F. **Strong bases** and **strong acids** are **totally dissociated** or ionized in solution; thus, they are **poorly absorbed at any pH.** Quaternary ammonium compounds are completely ionized at physiological pHs and therefore are also poorly absorbed.

G. Many routes of drug administration can be used.

  1. The **oral route** (PO) is usually preferred.

    a. Advantages include:

    (1) Convenience

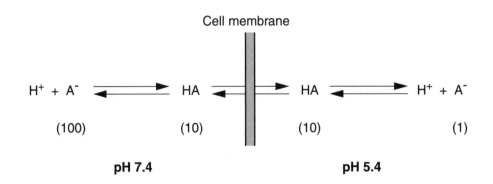

Figure 1-1. Ion trapping of a weak acid (pK_a 6.4) on the side of the cell membrane with the higher pH. The numbers in parentheses represent the relative concentrations of each form of the weak acid under steady state conditions.

       (2) A **large surface area** for absorption

       (3) Less abrupt changes of serum drug concentrations than with parenteral administration

     b. A **major disadvantage is first pass metabolism** by the liver.

       (1) All the blood flow from the intestinal tract goes initially to the liver through the portal vein; therefore, the **drug may be metabolized before being distributed** to the other tissues in the body.

       (2) First pass metabolism of a drug can be **avoided by sublingual administration** and partially avoided by rectal administration.

  2. The **parenteral routes** of administration are technically more difficult and usually must be performed by a health care professional.

     a. Advantages include:

       (1) A faster onset (usually)

       (2) More reliable absorption

       (3) No first pass metabolism

     b. Disadvantages include:

       (1) More difficult administration

       (2) Pain or necrosis at the site of injection

       (3) Possibility of **infection**

       (4) Toxicity from a bolus intravenous (IV) injection

       (5) Necessity of dissolving the drug if given intravenously

H. The **initial distribution** of a drug to the tissues is determined by the **relative blood flows** to the tissues. Sites with high blood flows will initially receive more of the drug.

I. The final distribution, also called the **apparent volume of distribution (V_d),** will be affected by:

  1. The lipid solubility of a drug, which, if high, will result in good penetration into cells and a high V_d.

  2. Plasma protein binding and tissue binding

     a. Plasma protein binding, especially to albumin, will reduce the V_d.

     b. Tissue binding will increase the V_d.

     c. Both types of binding act as **reservoirs** for the drug, as only the unbound drug can activate pharmacological receptors. Thus binding will:

       (1) Slow the onset of drug action

       (2) Prolong the duration of drug action, if the drug is eliminated by glomerular filtration in the kidney

II. METABOLISM OF DRUGS

A. The **liver** is the **primary site of drug metabolism.**

B. Metabolism can change a drug in several ways.

  1. The **polarity is usually increased,** enhancing the water solubility and renal excretion of the drug metabolite.

  2. The **activity of the drug is reduced. Exceptions** are the **prodrugs,** which are drugs that are inactive in the form administered but are metabolized to their active forms.

  3. A drug metabolite usually has a **smaller V_d.**

C. Phase 1 metabolic reactions lead to the **degradation** of the drug.

  1. Oxidation by mixed function oxidases (MFO) [also known as cytochrome P450s, microsomal enzymes, mono-oxygenases] **occurs** in the **smooth endoplasmic reticulum (ER).**

    a. Nicotinamide adenine dinucleotide phosphate (NADPH), **cytochrome P450 reductase,** and elemental oxygen **(O_2)** are required.

    b. Many reactions can be produced, including:

        (1) Hydroxylation

        (2) Dealkylation

        (3) Deamination

        (4) Sulfoxidation

        (5) Oxidation

    c. Highly lipid soluble drugs are more readily metabolized by MFOs.

  2. Reductive reactions can occur in the ER or the cytosol.

  3. Hydrolytic reactions do not occur in the ER.

D. Phase 2 metabolic reactions are **conjugative** (synthetic).

  1. Glucuronidation occurs in the **ER.** Glucose is used to form uridine diphosphate glucuronic acid (UDPGA) which then transfers a glucuronide to the drug in the presence of glucuronyl transferase.

  2. Other substances can be conjugated (by transferases primarily in the cytosol) to drugs, thereby reducing the drug activity, including:

    a. Sulfate

    b. Acetyl

    c. Methyl

    d. Glutathione

    e. Amino acids, especially glycine

E. Many drug **interactions** are due to changes in MFO (cytochrome P450s) activity in the liver.

  1. Induction of MFOs results from increased levels of MFOs in the ER.

    a. The onset of induction is **slow** (days) and the duration is **long** (taking a week or more for recovery).

    b. Many drugs that are metabolized by the MFOs also induce the MFOs, including

        (1) Barbiturates, phenytoin, rifampin, warfarin

        (2) Alcohol

        (3) Cigarette smoke

    c. This induction hastens the metabolism of the inducing drug and many other drugs.

  2. Inhibition of drug metabolism occurs if there is **competition** between drugs at the MFO, or if a drug tightly binds to the MFO, e.g., **cimetidine.** Grapefruit juice has a similar inhibitory effect.

III. EXCRETION OF DRUGS AND DRUG METABOLITES

A. The **kidney** is the primary organ that excretes drugs and drug metabolites.

  1. If the drug is excreted in the unmetabolized form, the kidney also decreases the pharmacological activity.

  2. Polar drugs and **polar drug metabolites** are readily eliminated by the kidney.

B. Filtration of the unbound molecule accounts for the excretion of most drugs.

  1. Drug molecules bound by plasma proteins will not be filtered by the glomerulus.

  2. Hydrophilic or lipophobic substances are most **efficiently eliminated** by the kidney, because they are not readily reabsorbed across the nephron tubule after they are filtered.

3. If a drug is a **weak base,** administration of ammonium chloride will **acidify the urine** and increase the amount of the base that is in the ionized form.
  a. The **excretion of the weak base will be increased.**
  b. This will be most effective if the pK_a of the drug is near the physiological pH.

4. The **excretion of a weak acid can be increased by alkalinizing the urine** with sodium bicarbonate.

C. Active transport of a few drugs occurs in the **proximal tubule.**

  1. It usually involves **secretion of strong acids or strong bases.**

  2. P-glycoprotein functions as an important transporter in renal and other cells.

  3. Characteristics of active transport are:
    a. **Competition** between substrates for the carrier
    b. **Saturation** of the carrier
    c. **Being unaffected by plasma protein binding**

  4. Active reabsorption can also occur.

  5. A few substances are both actively secreted and actively reabsorbed (e.g., uric acid, aspirin).

D. Biliary excretion occurs in the liver.

  1. Large polar compounds, often conjugated metabolites, are actively excreted into the bile.

  2. Enterohepatic cycling occurs with a few drugs that are eliminated in the bile, re-absorbed from the intestine, returned to the liver and again eliminated in the bile.
    a. Glucuronidase in the intestine can cleave off the glucuronide, so the free drug can be reabsorbed (Figure 1–2).
    b. Digitoxin, a cardiac glycoside, undergoes enterohepatic cycling.
    c. This may increase the half-life of the drug.

IV. CLINICAL PHARMACOKINETICS

A. Clinical pharmacokinetics, which involves the **mathematical description** of the **processes of drug absorption, distribution, metabolism,** and **elimination,** is useful to predict the serum drug concentrations under various conditions.

B. **Absorption of a drug is usually fast,** as compared to the elimination; thus, it is often ignored in kinetic calculations.

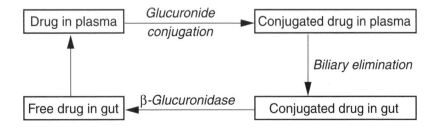

Figure 1-2. Enterohepatic cycling of a conjugated drug.

C. Elimination usually follows the principles of **first-order kinetics,** which means that a constant fraction of the drug is eliminated per unit of time (K_e).

D. Several **equations** are useful.

1. Bioavailability (F) equation:

$$F = \frac{\text{concentration of drug in the systemic circulation after oral administration}}{\text{concentration of drug in the systemic circulation after IV administration}}$$

a. The **bioavailability** after oral administration depends on:
(1) The **disintegration** of a tablet
(2) The **dissolution** of the drug in the intestinal contents
(3) Gastrointestinal and **first-pass metabolism**
b. **Bioequivalence** occurs when drugs with equal F have the same drug concentration versus time relationship.

2. Apparent volume of distribution equation:

$$V_d = \frac{\text{amount of drug injected}}{\text{serum [drug]}}$$

a. The V_d is an approximation of a volume that a drug appears to distribute in. It can be very large, even larger than the total body volume, if a drug is highly bound to tissues. This makes the serum drug concentration very low and the V_d very large.
b. The V_d must be calculated at the time of injection.
c. For the drugs illustrated in Figure 1–3, if the same amount of each was administered, the concentration of drug A at time 0 will be lower; thus, it will have the larger V_d.

3. The **loading dose** for a drug is based on the V_d.

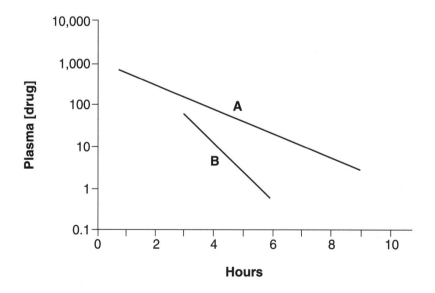

Figure 1-3. Relationship of plasma drug concentration versus time for two drugs. Drug A has the larger apparent volume of distribution.

$$\text{Oral loading dose} = \frac{V_d \times C}{F}$$

where C is the desired or target serum drug concentration.

4. Clearance (Cl) equals $V_d \times K_e$
   a. Clearance is measured as a volume per unit of time.
   b. The rate of drug elimination equals $Cl \times C_{ss}$, where C_{ss} is the drug concentration at steady state.
   c. The **oral maintenance dose** simply involves the replacement of the amount of drug that has been eliminated in the dosage interval (T)

$$\text{Oral maintenance dose} = \frac{Cl \times C_{ss} \times T}{F}$$

5. The **half-life** ($t_{1/2}$) of a drug is the time required for the serum drug concentration to be reduced by 50%.

   a. $t_{1/2} = \dfrac{0.69}{K_e}$

   b. If the $t_{1/2}$ of a drug is 5 hours, then the serum drug concentration will be reduced by 75% in 10 hours.
   c. During repeated administrations, it takes **4 to 5 half-lives to attain a steady state drug concentration.**
   d. When the dosage interval (T) is reduced with the same total amount of drug being administered, the $t_{1/2}$ is not changed.
      (1) The fluctuations of the drug concentration become smaller.
      (2) This is a useful approach when a drug has a very narrow therapeutic window between the effective drug concentration and the toxic drug concentration.

6. With **reduced kidney function,** the maintenance dose should be reduced if the drug is cleared from the body by the kidney.

   a. Oral maintenance dose $= \dfrac{(Cl_{hepatic} + Cl_{renal} + Cl_{others}) \times C_{ss} \times T}{F}$

   b. **Creatinine clearance** is a good quantitative **indicator of glomerular filtration rate.** Serum creatinine may also serve as a useful index of glomerular filtration rate.

7. With **reduced liver function,** there is **no good predictor** of the oral maintenance dose for drugs that are cleared by the liver.
   a. If the **extraction ratio** for a drug passing through the liver **approaches 1,** then Cl equals hepatic blood flow (BF).
      (1) **Reduced hepatic BF or reduced cardiac output (CO) will reduce the hepatic Cl of a drug with a high hepatic extraction ratio.**
      (2) An example is **lidocaine,** which has a lower $Cl_{hepatic}$ in patients with congestive heart failure. As a result, the maintenance dose of lidocaine should be reduced in these patients.
   b. If the hepatic extraction ratio is near 0, hepatic BF is unimportant. Intrinsic metabolic rate and the amount of plasma protein binding become important factors.

8. If a drug follows first-order elimination kinetics, **doubling the dose will double the** C_{ss}.

E. The above equations **do not apply** to drugs that have **zero-order** elimination kinetics (i.e., those for which a constant amount of drug is eliminated per unit of time).

   1. It is very difficult to predict and control the C_{ss} for these drugs.

   2. Drugs which follow zero-order kinetics include:
   a. Ethanol
   b. Heparin
   c. Phenytoin
   d. Aspirin at high concentrations

V. PEDIATRIC PHARMACOLOGY

A. Newborns have **more body water and less body fat** than adults.

   1. A **water-soluble drug will have a higher** V_d (relative to body size) in children than in adults.

   2. A **lipid-soluble drug will have a lower** V_d (relative to body size) in children than in adults.

B. **Plasma protein binding is reduced** for approximately the first year.

C. **Metabolism,** especially oxidation and glucuronidation, is also **reduced**.

D. **Glomerular filtration rate (GFR) and renal tubular function** are **reduced** in newborns.

VI. GERIATRIC PHARMACOLOGY

A. The **elderly** generally have:

   1. A **smaller** body mass

   2. **More body fat** and less body water
   a. A water soluble drug will have a lower V_d than in a person of average age.
   b. A lipid soluble drug will have a higher V_d.

   3. **Reduced plasma albumin,** which will reduce the amount of bound drug in the plasma

   4. **Reduced renal excretion**

   5. **Reduced hepatic metabolism** of some drugs

   6. Other non-pharmacokinetic changes
   a. Central nervous system (CNS) drugs often produce confusion.
   b. Cardiovascular drugs often have greater effects in the elderly patient because the homeostatic mechanisms (e.g., baroreceptor reflexes) are sluggish.

B. Overall, elderly patients require smaller dosages of most drugs than young adults.

VII. PHARMACODYNAMICS

A. **Pharmacodynamics** is a description of the properties of **drug-receptor interactions.**

B. **Drugs bind** to specific receptors with:

   1. Ionic bonds

   2. Hydrogen bonds

   3. Van der Waals forces, which are weak but necessary for a good fit

   4. Covalent bonds, which are uncommon and are usually irreversible

C. **Agonists** change the effector site and **lead to drug effects.**

    1. The drug-receptor interaction follows the **laws of mass action.**

        a. Drug molecules bind to receptors at a rate that is dependent on the drug concentration.

        b. The number of drug-receptor interactions determines the magnitude of the drug effect.

    2. This leads to **dose–response** curves, which can be:

        a. **Quantal** (all or none) [e.g., death]

        b. **Graded** (e.g., blood pressure)

D. The **therapeutic index** (TI) is a measure of the **safety** of a drug. (Figure 1–4)

$$TI = \frac{LD_{50}}{ED_{50}}$$

    1. LD_{50} is the dose that kills 50% of the subjects.

    2. ED_{50} is the dose that produces the desired effect in 50% of the subjects.

E. Other indexes can be used, including:

    1. $\dfrac{LD_1}{ED_{99}}$

    2. $\dfrac{TD_{50}}{ED_{50}}$, where TD_{50} is the dose that induces a toxic effect in 50% of the subjects.

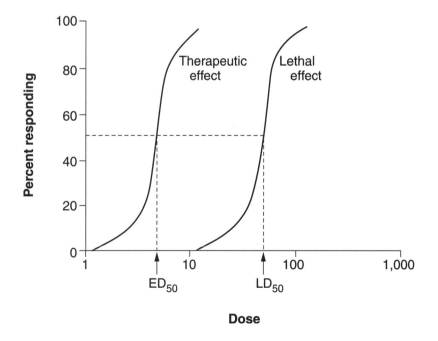

Figure 1-4. Dose-response relationships for a therapeutic effect and the lethal effect of a drug. The distance between these curves is indicative of the safety of the drug and the TI is approximately 10. ED_{50} = effective dose in 50% of patients; LD_{50} = lethal dose in 50% of patients

F. The **potency** (affinity) of a drug is inversely related to the ED_{50}.

G. The **intrinsic activity** (efficacy) is equivalent to the **maximal effect.**

   1. In Figure 1–5, drug B has the higher intrinsic activity.

   2. Drug A (see Figure 1–5) is approximately 10 times more potent than drug B, because the ED_{50} of drug A is 10% the ED_{50} of drug B.

   3. Drug A is a partial agonist (or a partial antagonist), because the maximal response is smaller.

H. **Antagonists** are drugs with a high affinity for a receptor and **no intrinsic activity.** They alter the dose-response curves for the agonists.

   1. **Competitive surmountable** (reversible) antagonists induce a **parallel shift** of the agonist dose-response curve to the right with no change in intrinsic activity (Figure 1–6A). In other words, the effect of the antagonist can be surmounted by increasing the concentration of the agonist.

   2. The **maximal effect** of a specific agonist **is reduced** (increasing the concentration of the agonist will not surmount the effect of the antagonist) with little or no change in the ED_{50} of the agonist (Figure 1–6B) by:

     a. **Competitive insurmountable (irreversible) antagonists,** which often bind covalently to a receptor

     b. **Non-competitive antagonists,** which often act at a site other than the receptor for the agonist

I. **Other types of antagonism** can occur.

   1. **Functional** (physiological) antagonism involves the opposing actions of **2 agonists** at different receptors [e.g., acetylcholine (ACh) and norepinephrine (NE) on heart rate].

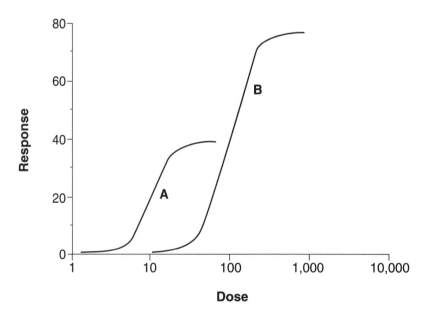

Figure 1-5.   Dose-response relationships for two drugs. Drug B has the higher intrinsic activity. Drug A is approximately 10 times more potent than Drug B.

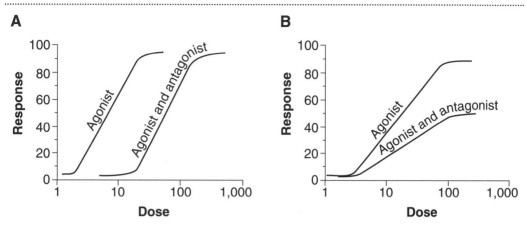

Figure 1-6.   Dose-response relationships for an agonist alone and for an agonist in the presence of (A) a competitive surmountable antagonist and (B) a competitive insurmountable or non-competitive antagonist.

Table 1-1
Procedures for Development of New Drugs (established by Kefauver-Harris Amendment, 1962)

---

1. **Animal studies** are initially performed to determine the activity and toxicity in more than one species.
2. An **IND application** is submitted to the FDA.
3. The **clinical phases** are begun.
   * **Phase 1** involves studies of kinetics in approximately 10 healthy volunteers.
   * **Phase 2** involves studies of the dosage range, effectiveness, and toxicity in approximately 100 patients, utilizing single or double-blind methods.
   * **Phase 3** involves studies of the same parameters in approximately 1000 patients. Special attention is paid to toxicities with low frequencies.
   * The **NDA** must be approved by the FDA.
   * **Phase 4** (NDA Phase) is a monitored release of the new drug to many physicians to detect rare toxicities.

FDA=Food and Drug Administration; *IND*=Investigational New Drug; *NDA*=New Drug Application

2. **Chemical antagonism** involves the **direct binding** of a drug by another drug without the involvement of a receptor (e.g., heavy metal chelators).

VIII. REGULATIONS GOVERNING THE DEVELOPMENT OF NEW DRUGS

A. In 1962, the **Kefauver-Harris Amendment to the Food, Drug and Cosmetic Act of 1938** was passed, as a result of thalidomide toxicity that occurred in Europe.

    1. The **Food and Drug Administration (FDA)** was charged with regulating drugs.

    2. **Procedures** were developed **for testing** new drugs. The procedures include animal studies, an Investigational New Drug (IND) application, human studies, and a New Drug Application (NDA) (Table 1–1).

B. The **ANDA** (Abbreviated NDA) was established so that it is only necessary to demonstrate bioequivalence for a generic form of an approved drug.

C. **Prescriptions** are required to dispense drugs that are:

1. **In the NDA Phase** of development

2. **Toxic**

3. **Habit-forming.** These drugs are divided into schedules based on their **potential for abuse,** as required by the Controlled Substances Act of 1970.
   a. **Schedule C-I drugs** are drugs of abuse with **no clinical use.**
   b. The others are **clinically useful.**
      (1) **Schedule C-II** drugs are highly abused.
      (2) **Schedule C-III** drugs are less commonly abused.
      (3) **Schedule C-IV** drugs are even less commonly abused.
      (4) **Schedule C-V** drugs have minor potential for abuse and may even be available over-the-counter.

2

Peripheral Neuropharmacology

I. OVERVIEW OF THE AUTONOMIC NERVOUS SYSTEM

A. This part of the peripheral nervous system **regulates the activity of cardiac muscle, smooth muscle,** and **exocrine glands.** It has two major divisions.

1. The **parasympathetic nervous system** refers to the division of the autonomic nervous system arising from the **brainstem** and the **sacral region** of the spinal cord.
   a. **Acetylcholine (ACh)** is the neurotransmitter at **both the ganglionic and neuroeffector synapses** (Figure 2–1).
   b. The **receptors** activated by ACh in the ganglion are **nicotinic (N) cholinoceptors,** and those in the neuroeffector junction are **muscarinic (M) cholinoceptors.**

2. The **sympathetic nervous system** refers to the division of the autonomic nervous system arising from the **thoracic and lumbar** regions of the spinal cord.
   a. **ACh** is the neurotransmitter in the **ganglionic synapse;** and **norepinephrine (NE)** is the neurotransmitter at the **neuroeffector synapse. Exceptions** include:
      (1) N-cholinergic innervation of the **adrenal medulla**
      (2) Sympathetic M-cholinergic innervation of some **sweat glands**
      (3) Sympathetic M-cholinergic innervation of some **muscle blood vessels**
      (4) Sympathetic dopaminergic innervation of **renal blood vessels**
   b. The **receptors** in the ganglion are **N-cholinoceptors** and those at the neuroeffector junction are **α- and β-adrenoceptors.**

B. The **synthesis and breakdown** of the **neurotransmitters** in the autonomic nervous system have been determined.

1. **ACh** is synthesized in the nerve terminal from **choline and acetyl coenzyme A in the presence of choline acetyltransferase.** After it is released, the ACh is broken down to choline and acetate by cholinesterases.

2. **NE synthesis** involves many steps (Figure 2–2).
   a. **Tyrosine hydroxylase** is the **rate-limiting step** in the synthesis and is also the **site for negative feedback inhibition** by NE.
   b. **Dopamine (DA)** is taken up into the granule and **metabolized by the granular enzyme, DA β-hydroxylase.**
   c. NE is complexed to adenosine triphosphate (ATP) and chromogranins in the granule.
   d. **Sites where epinephrine (EPI) is a neurotransmitter** have a **methyltransferase** that **converts NE to EPI.**
   e. The **NE** that is released **can be taken back up into the nerve ending (reuptake),** it can be **metabolized,** or it can **diffuse away from the synapse.**

Parasympathetic transmitters (cranial and sacral)

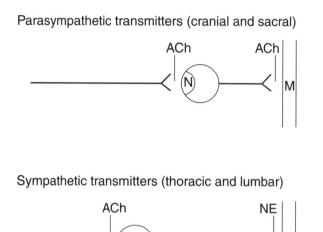

Sympathetic transmitters (thoracic and lumbar)

Figure 2-1. Neurotransmitters in the parasympathetic and sympathetic nervous systems. N = nicotinic cholinoceptors, M = muscarinic cholinoceptors, α = α-adrenoceptors, β = β-adrenoceptors. ACh=acetylcholine; NE=norepinephrine

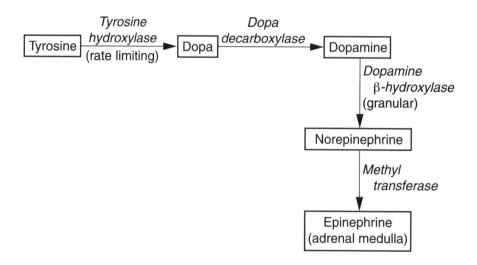

Figure 2-2. Synthesis of norepinephrine.

(1) **Reuptake** is the most important mechanism for the termination of NE action.

(2) **Cocaine** or **tricyclic antidepressants block the reuptake** of NE, thereby enhancing the neurotransmitter effects.

   f. **Catechol-O-methyltransferase (COMT) and monoamine oxidase (MAO)** convert NE to a final product, **methoxyhydroxymandelic acid (vanillylmandelic acid)** that **accounts for 90% of the NE and NE metabolites found in the urine** (Figure 2–3).

  C. The **effects of sympathetic and parasympathetic nerve stimulation** are listed in Table 2–1. Many of the effects of the autonomic drugs can be predicted from a thorough understanding of this table.

Table 2-1
Effects of Autonomic Nerve Activity on Organ Function

Organ	Sympathetic Nerve Activity	Parasympathetic Nerve Activity
Eye	α-contracts radial muscle (mydriasis) —	M-contracts circular muscle (miosis) M-contracts ciliary muscle
Heart	β_1-accelerates SA node β_1-accelerates conduction β_1-increases contractility	M-decelerates SA node M-decelerates conduction —
Vascular smooth muscle	α-constricts skin, skeletal muscle and splanchnic vessels β_2-dilates skeletal muscle vessels M-dilates skeletal muscle vessels (minor) DA-dilates renal and mesenteric vessels	—M(+)
Bronchiolar smooth muscle	β_2-dilates bronchioles	M-constricts bronchioles
Gastrointestinal tract	β_2-reduces gut contractility α-contracts sphincters —	M-increases gut contractility M-relaxes sphincters M-increases secretions
Genitourinary tract	β_2-reduces bladder motility α-contracts sphincters β_2-relaxes the pregnant uterus α-contracts the uterus α-ejaculation	M-increases bladder motility M-relaxes sphincters — — M-penile erection
Skin	α-contracts pilomotor smooth muscle M-induces sweating	— —
Metabolic functions	α, β_2-increases hepatic gluconeogenesis α, β_2-increases hepatic glycogenolysis β_3-increases lipolysis	— — —
Glands	α_1-thick salivary secretions —	M-thin salivary secretions M-lacrimal and respiratory secretions
Adrenal gland	N-secretes EPI and NE	—
Kidney	β_1-increases renin release	—

+ Most blood vessels have uninnervated muscarinic cholinoceptors. Relaxation involves release of endothelium-derived relaxing factor (EDRF) from the endothelium.
α=α-adrenoceptors; β=β-adrenocepters; *DA*=dopamine; *EPI*=epinephrine; *M*=muscarinic cholinoceptors; *N*=nicotinic cholinoceptors; *NE*=nonepinephrine; *SA*=sinoatrial; — = no effect

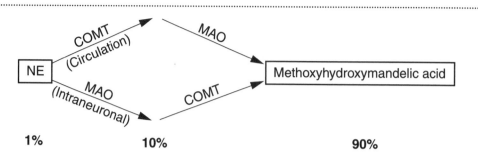

Figure 2-3. Metabolism of norepinephrine by catechol-O-methyl transferase (COMT) and monoamine oxidase (MAO). The percentages represent the proportions of each form found in the urine. *NE*=norepinephrine

II. PARASYMPATHOMIMETICS

A. Drugs in this class produce effects similar to activation of the parasympathetic nervous system.

B. Specific drugs

1. **ACh** acts at **N-cholinoceptors** and **M-cholinoceptors.**
   a. There are **2 binding sites** for ACh on the ACh receptors. One binds the **quaternary nitrogen** and the second binds the **carbonyl oxygen** (Figure 2–4).
   b. ACh has some major **disadvantages.**
      (1) It **activates all cholinoceptors, which are present in most internal organs,** leading to **many side effects** from administration.
      (2) It has a **short duration of action** due to rapid metabolism by cholinesterases.

2. **Analogues of ACh** are available that have slightly different properties than ACh (Table 2–2)
   a. All of these are **quaternary ammonium** compounds.
   b. **Carbachol** and **bethanechol** have **greater effects on the gastrointestinal** and **urinary tracts** and **longer durations of action** than ACh and methacholine.

3. **Two alkaloids** have parasympathomimetic activity.
   a. **Muscarine** is a **quaternary amine** that acts only on muscarinic receptors.
   b. **Pilocarpine** is a **tertiary amine** that acts only on muscarinic receptors.
      (1) As a tertiary amine, it is **more readily absorbed.**
      (2) It **penetrates the blood-brain barrier** to reach the CNS.
      (3) It is very effective at enhancing salivary secretions.

C. The effects of all the parasympathomimetics are **similar to the effects of parasympathetic nerve stimulation** (see Table 2–1).

1. The parasympathomimetics also **activate uninnervated cholinoceptors** (e.g., M-cholinoceptors in blood vessels to lower blood pressure) and M-cholinoceptors at sympathetic cholinergic synapses.

2. The dilating effect of parasympathomimetics **on blood vessels is mediated by the release of endothelium-derived relaxing factor (EDRF),** which is probably nitric oxide, from the endothelium. An intact endothelium is required for these effects to occur.

3. An **overdose** of a parasympathomimetic leads to:
   a. **A marked fall in blood pressure**

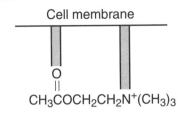

Cell membrane

$$CH_3COCH_2CH_2N^+(CH_3)_3$$

Figure 2-4.   Binding of acetylcholine to the cholinoceptor. The two bars represent the binding sites on the receptor.

Table 2-2
Properties of ACh and ACh analogues

	Metabolized by cholinesterases	Nicotinic activity	GI activity	CV activity
ACh	+++	+	++	+++
Methacholine	+	⊖	+	+++
Carbachol	⊖	+	+++	+
Bethanechol (*Urecholine*)	⊖	⊖	+++	+

Note: unique features are circled
ACh=acetylcholine; *CV*=cardiovascular; *GI*=gastrointestinal

  b. **An increase in heart rate,** mediated via **reflexes** induced by the fall in blood pressure. The fall in blood pressure reduces afferent baroreceptor activity which leads to an increase in efferent sympathetic tone to the heart.
  c. Activation of M-cholinoceptors at many sites which induces a **DUMBELS syndrome,** composed of
   (1) Defecation
   (2) Urination
   (3) Miosis
   (4) Bronchoconstriction
   (5) Emesis
   (6) Lacrimation
   (7) Salivation
 D. The **clinical uses** of the parasympathomimetics are **limited.**
  1. **Gastrointestinal (GI) atony and bladder atony** can be treated with bethanechol.
  2. **Glaucoma** can be treated with pilocarpine (*Pilocar*).
  3. A **pupillary constriction** can be induced with pilocarpine.
  4. **Xerostomia** can be treated with pilocarpine (*Salagen*).
  5. A **diagnosis of atropine poisoning or asthma** can utilize methacholine.

III. CHOLINESTERASE INHIBITORS

 A. These drugs bind to and **inhibit acetylcholinesterases,** thereby **increasing the ACh concentration** in the cholinergic synapses.

1. Cholinesterase inhibitors are **indirect parasympathomimetics** because they **do not bind to ACh receptors.**

2. Butyrylcholinesterases (pseudocholinesterases) are also inhibited by the **cholinesterase inhibitors,** but the function of these cholinesterases is unknown.

3. The **characteristics of the important cholinesterase inhibitors** are summarized in Table 2–3 .

4. The mechanism of binding to cholinesterase varies, as **some bind both the esteratic (E) and anionic (A) sites,** and **some bind only one site** (See Table 2–3).

B. The **carbamates** and **edrophonium** are **reversible inhibitors** of cholinesterases.

C. The quaternary amines will not induce CNS effects because the quaternary structure precludes passage across the blood-brain barrier.

D. The **organophosphates** are **very lipid soluble** and are **irreversible inhibitors of cholinesterases.** This group includes

1. Diisopropyl phosphorofluoridate (DFP)

2. Echothiophate (*Phospholine*)

3. **Malathion** and **parathion**
  a. They must be metabolized to their active forms, **malaoxon** and **paraoxon.**
  b. They are more toxic to insects than to humans, because humans detoxify them more rapidly; thus they are effective as **insecticides.**

E. Effects

1. The effects of the cholinesterase inhibitors are primarily **muscarinic** in nature.
  a. A **DUMBELS** syndrome is induced.
  b. **Nicotinic effects** occur **only at high doses.**

2. An overdose of cholinesterase inhibitors causes **death** from **respiratory insufficiency.**
  a. The reduced respiratory function is due to
    (1) **Increased bronchial secretions**
    (2) **Bronchoconstriction**
    (3) **Central respiratory depression**
    (4) **Depolarizing neuromuscular blockade**
  b. The **specific antidotes** used for poisoning by the cholinesterase inhibitors are:
    (1) **Atropine at high dosages,** which blocks the muscarinic effects of the accumulated ACh.
    (2) **Pralidoxime (2-PAM)** (*Protopam*) which can **reactivate the cholinesterases** that have been inhibited by an organophosphate.

Table 2-3
Properties of Various Cholinesterase Inhibitors

Inhibitor	Binding sites	Chemical properties
Physostigmine (*Antilirium*)	E & A	Tertiary carbamate
Neostigmine (*Prostigmin*)	E & A	Quaternary carbamate
Pyridostigmine (*Mestinon*)	E & A	Quaternary carbamate
Edrophonium (*Tensilon*)	A	Quaternary (non-carbamate), short duration
Organophosphates	E	Irreversible

A=anionic; *E*=esteratic

(a) It **must be administered within a few hours after the exposure,** because an "aging" process occurs, and the organophosphate-cholinesterase complex becomes insensitive to 2-PAM.

(b) Pralidoxime will have **no effect on poisoning from the carbamates.**

3. Chronic exposure to the organophosphates leads to a **delayed neurotoxicity** due to **demyelinization of motor neurons.**

F. These drugs have many **clinical uses.**

   1. Paroxysmal supraventricular tachycardia (PSVT) can be terminated with edrophonium.

   2. Glaucoma can be reduced with echothiophate.

   3. Competitive neuromuscular blockade can be reversed with neostigmine.

     a. To **reduce the parasympathetic side effects of the cholinesterase inhibitors, atropine** should also be administered.

     b. Atropine has no effect on the skeletal neuromuscular junction, because there are no M-cholinoceptors at this site.

   4. Myasthenia gravis is treated with pyridostigmine.

   5. Myasthenia gravis can be diagnosed, and a **myasthenic crisis** can be differentiated from a **cholinergic crisis** with edrophonium.

   6. Alzheimer's disease can be somewhat reduced with tacrine (*Cognex*).

   7. Anticholinergic poisoning can be diagnosed and treated with cholinesterase inhibitors.

G. Contraindications for the use of cholinesterase inhibitors include:

   1. Asthma

   2. Peptic ulcers

IV. PARASYMPATHETIC BLOCKING DRUGS

A. Drugs in this class **block the effects of the parasympathetic nervous system.**

   1. Atropine is a **competitive, surmountable antagonist.**

     a. It blocks M_1, M_2, and M_3 cholinoreceptors.

     b. The **effects of ACh are reversed** (ACh reversal) by muscarinic antagonists.

       (1) The **muscarinic vasodilating actions** of ACh are **blocked.**

       (2) The **nicotinic (ganglion) vasoconstricting actions** from high doses of ACh are **unmasked.**

   2. Scopolamine is similar to atropine, except there are more CNS effects, which may occur even at therapeutic doses.

   3. Both are **tertiary amines,** so they will penetrate into the CNS.

B. The **effects, uses,** and **side effects** are summarized in Table 2–4. Note that atropine will not increase blood pressure because there is no parasympathetic tone to the blood vessels.

C. Both anticholinergics and phenylephrine, an α_1-adrenoceptor agonist, induce mydriasis, but **phenylephrine will not induce cycloplegia** (loss of accommodation).

D. These drugs have a **large therapeutic index.**

   1. Hallucinations can be induced.

Table 2-4
Effects, Uses, and Side Effects of the Parasympathetic Blocking Drugs

Effects	Uses	Side effects
Increase heart rate (may be an initial decrease due to vagal nuclei activity)	Bradycardia that is vagally mediated (e.g., digoxin therapy)	Tachycardia
Pupillary dilation and cycloplegia	Eye exam [tropicamide (*Mydriacyl*)]	Blurred vision Photophobia Angle closure glaucoma
Bronchodilation	Asthma [quarternary: ipratropium (*Atrovent*)]	
Decrease gut motility	Antispasmodic [propantheline (*Pro-Banthine*)]	Constipation
Decrease bladder contractions		Urinary retention
Decrease secretions	Preanesthetic medication	Dry mouth
Sedative	Preanesthetic medication	Drowsiness (scopolamine)
	Reduce motion sickness (scopolamine)	
	Parkinson's disease [trihexyphenidyl (*Artane*)]	
	Antagonize poisoning from cholinesterase inhibitors and muscarine	

2. High doses produce **life-threatening toxicity only in children,** who seem to be more sensitive to the drugs.

   a. The side effects in Table 2–4 will be accentuated.

   b. Hot skin and fever occur, due to a direct vasodilation.

3. Adult anticholinergic poisoning is more common with H_1 antihistamines, tricyclic antidepressants, and phenothiazines.

4. The antidote for anticholinergic poisoning is a **cholinesterase inhibitor** (e.g., physostigmine).

V. GANGLIONIC BLOCKING DRUGS

  A. Drugs in this class **competitively inhibit nicotinic cholinoceptors in the ganglion,** which leads to ganglionic blockade. These drugs have no effect on the neuromuscular nicotinic cholinoceptors.

    1. Hexamethonium and **trimethaphan** (*Arfonad*) are **polar amines.**

    2. Trimethaphan has a very short duration of action and is thus useful to treat hypertensive crises. Blockade of sympathetic ganglia by trimethaphan reduces peripheral vascular resistance and lowers blood pressure.

  B. The **major limitation** of the ganglionic blocking drugs is that they **inhibit both sympathetic and parasympathetic ganglia.**

    1. This results in **many autonomic side effects.**

    2. Less toxic drugs are available for the treatment of **essential hypertension.**

  C. When both sympathetic and parasympathetic ganglia are blocked by hexamethonium, the net effect will be equivalent to blockade of the dominant autonomic system for each tissue.

D. Nicotine activates nicotinic receptors at:

1. Sensory nerve endings

2. Ganglia

3. Adrenal medulla

4. Neuromuscular junction, leading to depolarization block

VI. SYMPATHOMIMETICS

A. Drugs in this class **mimic the effects of the sympathetic nervous system** by activating adrenoceptors or inducing the release of endogenous NE.

B. There are 2 groups of sympathomimetics.

1. **Catecholamines** have a **catechol** (3,4 dihydroxybenzine) in the structure (Figure 2–5).

    a. The *l*-form is active.

    b. **Administration by parenteral injection or inhalation** is used because of rapid metabolism in the gut and first-pass metabolism.

    c. Important **catecholamines** are:

        (1) NE, an α and β_1 agonist

        (2) EPI, an α, β_1 and β_2 agonist

        (3) Isoproterenol (Iso), a β_1 and β_2 agonist

        (4) Dobutamine (*Dobutrex*), a β_1 agonist

        (5) DA, which:

            (a) Is an agonist at **DA receptors (renal and mesenteric vasodilator)** at low doses

            (b) Is an **indirect agonist** and a β_1 **agonist (myocardial stimulant)** at intermediate doses

            (c) Is an α **agonist (vasoconstrictor)** at high doses

2. **Phenylethylamines** do not have the catechol structure and thus are **less readily metabolized** and **more effective when given orally.**

    a. **Phenylephrine** (*Neo-Synephrine*) and methoxamine (*Vasoxyl*) are α_1 agonists.

    b. **Clonidine** (*Catapres*) is an α_2 agonist.

    c. **Terbutaline** (*Bricanyl,Brethine*) **albuterol** (*Proventil,Ventolin*) and **ritodrine** (*Yutopar*) are β_2 **agonists.**

    d. **Tyramine** and the **amphetamines** are **indirect** sympathomimetics.

        (1) This means that they induce the release of endogeneous NE and it is the NE that activates the α- and β-adrenoceptors.

        (2) **Effects** of the indirect sympathomimetics will be **reduced by the following procedures.** The same procedures will not affect or will increase the effects of the direct sympathomimetics.

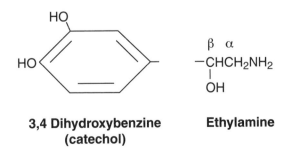

3,4 Dihydroxybenzine (catechol)   **Ethylamine**

Figure 2-5.   General structure of catecholamines, as illustrated with NE.

> **(a) Cocaine and tricyclic antidepressants** block the uptake of tyramine and NE into the adrenergic nerve ending, an action that reduces the effect of tyramine and augments the effects of exogenously administered NE.
>
> **(b) Denervation, reserpine, and guanethidine** deplete the endogenous catecholamines, thus the indirect agonists become ineffective and the effects of exogenous NE will be unchanged or enhanced.

C. The **cardiovascular effects** of each agonist will depend on the types of receptors that are activated.

1. NE, an α_1-agonist will induce (Figure 2–6):
  a. An **increase in blood pressure**
  b. A **reflex reduction in heart rate.** This indicates that the reflex baroreceptor effects are more important than the direct effects of NE on the heart. The reduction of heart rate can be blocked by atropine.

2. ISO, a β-agonist will induce (Figure 2–7):
  a. A **decrease in blood pressure (β_2)**
  b. **Large increases in heart rate and contractility,** due to both direct (β_1) and reflex effects.

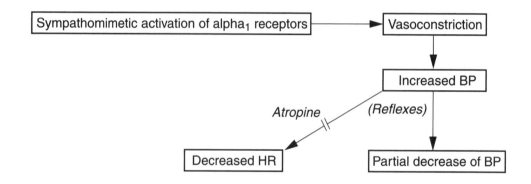

Figure 2-6. Effects of α-adrenoceptor activation on blood pressure and heart rate. The reflex effects on the heart (blocked by atropine) will predominate over the direct beta effects, if norepinephrine is the agonist.

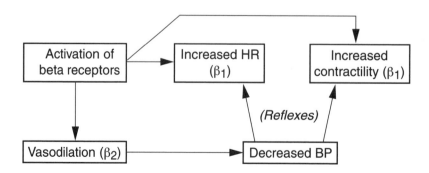

Figure 2-7. Effects of β-adrenoceptor activation on blood pressure and heart rate. Both the reflex and direct effects result in an increase in heart rate and contractility. *BP*=blood pressure; *HR*=heart rate

     3. EPI is an agonist at α, β_1 and β_2 adrenoceptors.

        a. At low doses it induces **little change of mean blood pressure** (α_1-vasoconstricting and β_2-vasodilating effects balance out), thus **heart rate will be increased due to direct β_1 effects on the heart.**

        b. At high doses, the α_1-vasoconstricting effect will predominate, mean blood pressure will increase, and heart rate will be reflexly reduced.

  D. Many of the effects of the catecholamines, especially the β-effects, are mediated by **activation of G-proteins** which leads to an increase in the second messenger, **cyclic adenosine monophosphate (cAMP).**

  E. The **effects, uses,** and **side effects** for the various sympathomimetics are summarized in Table 2–5.

VII. α-ADRENOCEPTOR ANTAGONISTS

  A. Drugs in this class **inhibit α-adrenoceptors,** thereby **reducing the α-effects of endogenously released NE.**

  B. Non-selective antagonists block both α_1- and α_2-adrenoceptors.

     1. The properties of the various α-antagonists are quite different.

        a. Phenoxybenzamine (*Dibenzyline*) is an **alkylating agent** due to the formation of a reactive intermediate.

          (1) A **covalent** (irreversible) interaction with α-receptors results in a **competitive, insurmountable antagonism.**

          (2) Phenoxybenzamine is very irritating when given subcutaneously or intramuscularly and therefore **can only be given orally** or **intravenously.**

Table 2-5
Effects, Uses, and Side Effects from Activation of Adrenergic Receptors

Receptors	Effects	Uses	Side effects
α	Vasoconstriction	Hypotension Nasal congestion Reduce bleeding PSVT (phenylephrine) Prolong local anesthesia (EPI)	Hypertension Ischemia Bradycardia

β_2
β_1
	Vasodilation
	Increased myocardial
	  contractility
		Acute heart failure (Iso and
		  dobutamine)
			Coronary insufficiency
			Palpitations

β_1	Increased myocardial conduction	Heart block	Tachycardia Arrhythmias
β_2	Bronchodilation	Anaphylactic shock (EPI) Asthma (Iso, terbutaline and albuterol)	Muscle tremor
DA	Dilated renal and mesenteric vessels	Cardiogenic shock (DA)	

β_2
α
	Uterine relaxation
	Mydriasis without
	  cycloplegia
	Reduced intraocular
	  pressure
		Premature labor (ritodrine)
		Eye exam (phenylephrine)
		
		Glaucoma (EPI)	

DA=dopamine; *EPI*=epinephrine; *Iso*=isoproterenol; *PVST*=paroxysmal supraventricular tachycardia

    b. Phentolamine (*Regitine*) is a **competitive, surmountable antagonist.**
        (1) The **duration of action is short.**
        (2) It is effective after oral or parenteral administration.
    c. Ergot alkaloids are α-antagonists, vasoconstrictors, and oxytocics.
        (1) Ergotoxine is the most potent **α-antagonist.**
        (2) Ergotamine is the most potent **vasoconstrictor.** The vasoconstriction is unrelated to autonomic receptor actions.
        (3) Ergonovine is the most potent **oxytocic.**

2. When EPI is administered IV in the presence of an α-antagonist, the **normal pressor effect of EPI is reversed to a depressor effect.**
    a. α-Receptor activation by EPI, which normally increases blood pressure, is blocked.
    b. β_2-Receptor activation by EPI leads to a drop of blood pressure.

3. The effect of NE on blood pressure is inhibited, but not reversed, by the α-antagonists, because NE has much weaker β-agonistic effects than EPI.

4. The clinical **uses** of phenoxybenzamine and phentolamine are limited.
    a. **Pheochromocytoma** can be diagnosed and treated.
    b. **Peripheral vascular disease** can be treated.
    c. Blood pressure is reduced, but not by very much; thus they are **not used to treat essential hypertension.** Also, **side effects** are more common than with other anti-hypertensive drugs.
        (1) **Postural hypotension** results from:
            (a) **Venule dilation**
            (b) **Impaired sympathetic reflexes** to the blood vessels
        (2) **Tachycardia** results from increased sympathetic reflexes to the heart. This effect is enhanced by the α_2-blockade (blockade of presynaptic inhibitory sites), which leads to increased NE release and increased NE effects at sites where β-receptors predominate (e.g., myocardium).
        (3) **Renin release is increased.**

C. The newer drugs are **selective α-antagonists.**
    1. **Prazosin** (*Minipress*), **doxazosin** (*Cardura*) and **terazosin** (*Hytrin*) are selective **α_1-antagonists.**
        a. **Both arterioles and venules are dilated** leading to reduced preload and afterload on the heart.
        b. Blood pressure is reduced with less tachycardia and less renin release than with the non-selective antagonists.
        c. **Clinical indications** include:
            (1) **Essential hypertension**
            (2) **Prostatic hypertrophy**
        d. An important **side effect** is **first-dose syncope.**
    2. **Yohimbine** is a selective **α_2-antagonist** with no demonstrated clinical usefulness.

VIII. β-ADRENOCEPTOR ANTAGONISTS

A. Drugs in this class **inhibit β-adrenoceptors,** thereby **reducing the β-effects of endogenously released NE.**

B. β-Blockers are **structurally similar to the catecholamines.**
    1. They have **bulky alkyl** substitutions on the nitrogen and an **oxymethylene bridge** near the aromatic ring.
    2. The *l*-isomers are the active forms.

C. The non-selective β-blockers inhibit both β_1- and β_2-adrenoceptors.

   1. **Propranolol** (*Inderal*) is 90% bound to plasma proteins and is **rapidly metabolized by the liver.**

      a. The bioavailability is low (F = 0.3) due to first pass metabolism.

      b. The IV dose is one third of the oral dose.

      c. The half–life is short, approximately 3 hours.

      d. An active metabolite, hydroxypropranolol, is formed.

   2. The **effects, uses, side effects,** and **contraindications** of the β-blockers (e.g., propranolol) are listed in Table 2–6.

   3. Other **non-selective β-blockers** have important differences from propranolol.

      a. **Nadolol** (*Corgard*) is non-selective, water soluble and not metabolized, so the **half-life is long** (15 hours).

      b. **Pindolol** (*Visken*) is non-selective with **intrinsic sympathomimetic activity (ISA).**

         (1) It is a partial antagonist with β-agonistic activity.

         (2) Drugs with ISA induce less bradycardia.

      c. **Labetalol** (*Normodyne, Trandate*) and **carvedilol** (*Coreg*) are non-selective with α_1-**blocking activity.** They decrease blood pressure with less change of heart rate and contractility than other β-blockers.

D. Selective β_1-**blockers (cardioselective)** have weaker actions on the bronchi, making them more useful in patients with **asthma.** The β_1-selectivity is relative, however, so these drugs can still be dangerous when administered to asthmatics.

   1. **Metoprolol** (*Lopressor*) is β_1-selective.

Table 2-6
Effects, Uses, Side Effects, and Contraindications of Beta-Blockers

Effects	Uses	Side effects	Contraindications
Decreased heart rate	Tachycardia Angina Hyperthyroid crisis	Bradycardia	
Prolonged AV conduction time	Arrhythmias (e.g. PSVT)	Slow AV conduction	Heart block
Decreased myocardial contractility	Angina Mild heart failure	Heart failure	Severe heart failure
Bronchoconstriction Decreased glycogenolysis Peripheral vasoconstriction		Bronchospasm Hypoglycemia Vasoconstriction	Asthma Diabetes Peripheral vascular disease Angina at rest
Decreased blood pressure	Hypertension Glaucoma Migraine	CNS depression Insomnia Nightmares Sudden withdrawal can increase BP and induce arrhythmias Sexual dysfunction	

AV=atrioventricular; *BP*=blood pressure; *CNS*=central nervous system; *PSVT*=paroxysmal supraventricular tachycardia

2. Atenolol (*Tenormin*) is β_1-selective and **water soluble,** which results in **fewer CNS effects.**

3. Acebutolol (*Sectral*) is β_1-selective with **ISA.**

4. Esmolol (*Brevibloc*) is β_1-selective and is rapidly metabolized by esterases $(t_{1/2} = 9$ **minutes),** making it useful for emergency therapy.

IX. ADRENERGIC NEURON BLOCKING DRUGS

A. These drugs have **no effects on adrenergic receptors.** Instead, they **reduce the release of NE from the postganglionic adrenergic neuron.**

B. Reserpine (*Serpasil*) **depletes monoamines** [NE, DA and serotonin (5-HT)] and the depletion of NE results in sympathetic blockade, e.g. lowering of blood pressure.

    1. It acts by blocking the **granular catecholamine uptake.** Neuronal catecholamine uptake is unaffected.

    2. The **side effects** are very marked, including:

        a. Profound psychological depression and sedation. It must be used with caution when treating patients with a history of depression.

        b. Extrapyramidal symptoms from DA depletion

C. Guanethidine (*Ismelin*) is transported to the site of action in the nerve terminal via the neuronal catecholamine transport mechanism. The effects are **blocked by uptake inhibitors** (e.g., cocaine and tricyclic antidepressants).

    1. There is an **initial release of NE.**

    2. The **release is subsequently reduced** and depletion also occurs.

    3. The drug is very effective; but has **prominent side effects,** including:

        a. Symptoms of severe sympathetic block

        b. Severe postural hypotension

        c. Marked impotence

        d. Severe diarrhea

D. Several drugs **act on the CNS** to reduce the efferent sympathetic tone to the cardiovascular system.

    1. Methyldopa (*Aldomet*) is metabolized in CNS adrenergic neurons to α-**methyldopamine** and α-**methylnorepinephrine** (α-**methylNE).**

        a. α-**MethylNE** acts on α_2-adrenoceptors and decreases the sympathetic outflow from the medulla.

        b. The site of action appears to be the **nucleus tractus solitarius.**

    2. Clonidine (*Catapres*) and **guanabenz** (*Wytensin*) are α_2-**adrenoceptor agonists** that act like α-methylNE in the medulla.

    3. Side effects from the CNS active sympathetic blockers include:

        a. Drowsiness

        b. Fluid retention

        c. Positive Coombs' test (increased risk for hemolytic anemia) with **methyldopa**

        d. Acute withdrawal hypertension with clonidine

E. Bretylium (*Bretylol*) decreases NE release and is used for cardiac arrhythmias.

F. α-**Methyltyrosine** competitively **inhibits tyrosine hydroxylase,** and thereby depletes the NE. It is used to treat **pheochromocytoma,** if surgery is not possible.

X. DRUGS FOR GLAUCOMA

A. Open angle glaucoma is the most common type. It is treated with:

   1. Pilocarpine to **increase outflow** of intraocular fluid

   2. Timolol (*Timoptic*), a β-blocker, to **reduce the production** of intraocular fluid

   3. EPI to both increase outflow and reduce production of intraocular fluid

B. **Angle closure glaucoma** is induced when the iris dilates and obstructs the drainage of intraocular fluid. **Antimuscarinics,** which are pupillary dilators, can induce this type of glaucoma.

   1. Pilocarpine will **constrict the pupil** and lower the intraocular pressure.

   2. **Osmotic agents** will draw fluid from the eye.

   3. **Surgery** can correct the defect.

XI. NEUROMUSCULAR BLOCKING DRUGS

A. Drugs in this class **block skeletal neuromuscular transmission, thereby inducing a paralysis.**

B. **Competitive nicotinic antagonists** are **quaternary amines** that bind nicotinic cholinoceptors in the muscle end-plate region.

   1. The **end-plate potential (EPP) is reduced** below the threshold for the muscle action potential.

   2. The **safety factor** is approximately **5** at the neuromuscular junction, thus the EPP must be reduced to 20% of the normal amplitude for muscle paralysis to occur.
      a. A **reduction of the safety factor** and an increase in the sensitivity to competitive neuromuscular blocking drugs occurs with:
         (1) **Myasthenia gravis**
         (2) **General anesthetics,** which reduce the sodium and potassium permeability changes at the end-plate.
         (3) **Aminoglycoside antibiotics,** which reduce the release of ACh.
      b. An **increase in the safety factor** and a reversal of competitive neuromuscular blockade can be induced with the **cholinesterase inhibitors** (e.g., neostigmine).

   3. All the competitive neuromuscular blocking drugs act by the same mechanism, but they do have other properties that are different.
      a. *d*-Tubocurarine:
         (1) **Releases histamine,** which can lead to bronchospasm and lower blood pressure
         (2) **Blocks ganglionic nicotinic receptors,** which can also lower blood pressure
      b. **Pancuronium** (*Pavulon*) induces a vagal blockade which can increase heart rate and increase blood pressure.
      c. **Atracurium** (*Tracrium*) is very short acting.
      d. **Vecuronium** (*Norcuron*) has no cardiovascular side effects.

C. **Depolarizing** neuromuscular blocking drugs act like ACh. **Succinylcholine** (*Anectine*) is a quaternary amine.

   1. It binds to and **activates the nicotinic cholinoceptors.**
      a. The **events, leading to Phase 1 depolarization block,** are **initiated** (Figure 2–8).
      b. With long periods of paralysis, Phase 2 block characterized by receptor desensitization develops.

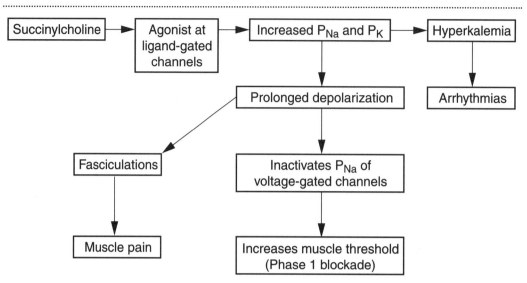

Figure 2-8.   Effects of depolarizing neuromuscular blocking drugs (e.g., succinylcholine). P_{Na}= sodium permeability. P_K=potassium permeability

2. Succinylcholine is **metabolized by butyrylcholinesterases** in the serum.
   a. **Succinylcholine apnea** can occur if a patient has a **genetic** defect that results in low butyrylcholinesterase activity.
      (1) **Excessive paralysis will be induced by a standard dose,** because less of the drug is metabolized before reaching the end-plate region.
      (2) **Paralysis of the respiratory muscles** (apnea) occurs with an over-dose.
   b. There is **no antidote** for succinylcholine paralysis.
      (1) Cholinesterase inhibitors will increase the paralysis by slowing the breakdown of succinylcholine and ACh.
      (2) Patients should be **ventilated** until the respiratory function returns.

3. The major advantage of succinylcholine is the **rapid onset and short duration** of paralysis.

D. The primary **uses** of neuromuscular blocking drugs are as an adjunct during **intubation** and for **muscle relaxation during surgery.**

E. Other drugs can affect muscle function by various mechanisms.

   1. **Hemicholinium** blocks the uptake of choline and leads to a depletion of ACh in the motor nerve terminal.

   2. **Botulinum toxin** (*Botox*) **blocks the release of ACh which induces a muscle paralysis.** It is used to reduce motor unit activity in eye and facial muscles.

   3. **α-Bungarotoxin** binds irreversibly to the neuromuscular nicotinic cholinoceptor.

   4. **Dantrolene** (*Dantrium*) **reduces calcium release from the sarcoplasmic reticulum** in skeletal muscle. This reduces the spasticity from **malignant hyperthermia** (e.g., as induced by inhalation anesthetics and neuromuscular blocking drugs).

   5. **Baclofen** (*Lioresal*) **is a central muscle relaxant that activates GABA$_B$ receptors** and thereby decreases spasticity.

XII. DRUGS FOR GASTROINTESTINAL DISORDERS

A. Ulcers can be treated in many ways.

    1. Triple antibiotic therapy (e.g., bismuth salts, tetracyclines, metronidazole ± omeprazole) will kill the *Helicobacter pylori* that causes the ulcers.

        a. A permanent **cure** can be produced in many patients.

        b. Antibiotic therapy is **inappropriate for salicylate-induced and nonsteroidal anti-inflammatory drug (NSAID)-induced ulcers.**

    2. H$_2$-**Antihistamines,** such as cimetidine (*Tagamet*), ranitidine (*Zantac*), and famotidine (*Pepcid*) are competitive antagonists at H$_2$-receptors in the intestinal tract.

        a. **Acid and pepsin secretion** are **reduced.**

        b. The release of intrinsic factor is unchanged.

        c. There are **no effects at H$_1$-receptors.**

        d. **Side effects** can occur.

            (1) Cimetidine:

                (a) Can cause **impotence** and **swelling of the breasts** due to antiandrogen activity.

                (b) **Increases prolactin release,** which can cause galactorrhea

                (c) **Inhibits mixed function oxidases,** which can slow the metabolism of many drugs (e.g., warfarin, propranolol) and enhance their effects.

            (2) **Ranitidine** and **famotidine** have **fewer side effects** and **longer durations** of action.

    3. Sucralfate (*Carafate*) adheres to the ulcerated mucosal wall of the stomach and provides a **barrier** to acid and pepsin.

    4. Omeprazole (*Prilosec*) **induces an irreversible inhibition of H$^+$/K$^+$ ATPase.**

        a. Acid secretion is decreased.

        b. It is very effective, especially for gastroesophageal reflux (heartburn).

    5. **Antacids directly neutralize stomach acid,** however their duration of action is limited by the stomach emptying time.

        a. **Sodium bicarbonate** is a **systemic** antacid.

            (1) It is readily absorbed into the body.

            (2) Side effects are common, including:

                (a) **Metabolic alkalosis**

                (b) **Hypernatremia**

                (c) **Fluid retention**

                (d) **Acid rebound,** due to high gastric pH

        b. **Non-systemic** antacids are poorly absorbed into the body.

            (1) **Magnesium hydroxide** induces the side effect of **diarrhea.**

            (2) **Aluminum hydroxide** induces **constipation.**

            (3) Magnesium hydroxide and aluminum hydroxide are frequently combined to create an antacid preparation with little effect on GI motility.

            (4) **Calcium carbonate** (*Tums*) has more **side effects,** including:

                (a) **Hypercalcemia** (e.g., milk alkali syndrome)

                (b) **Acid rebound**

                (c) **Constipation**

    6. Metoclopramide (*Octamide,Reglan*) is a **cholinomimetic** that **increases lower esophageal sphincter tone.**

        a. Gastroesophageal reflux is decreased.

        b. It also has anti-emetic actions.

    7. **Misoprostol** (*Cytotec*), a prostaglandin analogue, enhances the mucosal barrier and is used for **NSAID-induced** ulcers.

B. **Antidiarrheal drugs** are useful to reduce the loss of fluid and electrolytes that occurs with diarrhea. These drugs **should not be used for treating diarrhea that is caused by a poison, an infection, or chronic ulcerative colitis.**

   1. Opiates act by increasing the tone and reducing the motility of the GI tract.
      a. **Diphenoxylate,** which is insoluble and poorly absorbed, is combined **with atropine** (*Lomotil*).
      b. **Loperamide** (*Imodium*) has no systemic side effects.

   2. Antimuscarinics are ineffective for diarrhea, but will reduce the cramping from irritable bowel syndrome.

   3. **Attapulgite,** a hydrophilic substance, absorbs water and reduces the looseness of the feces.

C. **Laxative-cathartics** add bulk and water to the feces, thereby stimulating peristalsis and relieving constipation. They should **never be used for undiagnosed abdominal pain or when intestinal obstruction is possible.**

   1. Bulk laxatives (e.g., psyllium and methylcellulose) are **fiber,** which increases the volume of the GI contents and thereby enhances peristalsis.

   2. **Docusate** (*Colace, Doxinate*) is a **fecal softener** that makes the passage of stools easier.

   3. **Castor oil** and **bisacodyl** are contact laxatives.
      a. The active metabolite of castor oil is ricinoleic acid.
      b. **Irritation of nerve endings** increases peristaltic contractions.
      c. Prolonged use can lead to irritable bowel syndrome.

   4. **Osmotic (bulk) cathartics** are also called saline laxatives.
      a. **Magnesium sulfate** causes osmotic retention of large amounts of water in the gut.
      b. The increased bulk **markedly enhances peristalsis.**

3

Cardiovascular Pharmacology

I. DIURETICS

A. Drugs in this class act on the kidney to **enhance the elimination of salt and water** from the body.

B. Increased intake of water does increase urine volume, due to decreased antidiuretic hormone (ADH) and decreased renin release. Water is not a diuretic, however, because there is no net loss of body fluids.

C. **Ammonium chloride** induces a transient diuresis, and is useful only for:

  1. **Acidifying the urine** and increasing the elimination of weak bases

  2. **Treating metabolic alkalosis**

D. **Osmotic diuretics** [e.g., mannitol (*Osmitrol*), glycerol, urea] are **filtered by the kidney and not reabsorbed;** thus, these diuretics osmotically hold water in the tubules and increase urine flow. They can, however, increase extracellular volume, resulting in edema.

E. The **xanthines** (e.g., caffeine, theophylline, theobromine) produce a weak diuresis by increasing the glomerular filtration rate.

F. **Carbonic anhydrase inhibitors** [e.g., acetazolamide (*Diamox*)] **induce a bicarbonate loss** which leads to an alkaline diuresis.

G. **Thiazide** [e.g., hydrochlorothiazide (*Esidrix,HydroDIURIL*)] and thiazide-like [e.g. chlorthalidone (*Hygroton,Thalitone*)] diuretics act by **impairing the sodium and chloride cotransport** in the **initial part of the distal tubule.**

  1. The increased sodium in the tubular fluid holds water in the nephron, leading to the diuresis.

  2. The increased sodium in the tubular fluid also enhances Na^+/K^+ exchange, leading to a **hypokalemia.**

  3. The thiazides are effective when taken orally and are **eliminated by active proximal tubular secretion.**

  a. The secretion is important for the drugs to reach their intra-tubular site of action.

  b. Competition with the transport of uric acid at the same site can lead to hyperuricemia.

  4. **Side effects** from the thiazides include:

  a. **Hypokalemia,** which can increase the toxicity of the **cardiac glycosides**

  b. **Hyperuricemia**

    c. Hyperglycemia

    d. Small increases in low density lipoprotein (LDL) cholesterol

    e. Hypercalcemia

H. **Potassium-sparing diuretics** induce a weak diuresis by **reducing the sodium–potassium exchange** in the **late portion of the distal tubule and collecting ducts.** The serum potassium is elevated as a result of this action.

    1. **Spironolactone** (*Aldactone*) is a **competitive aldosterone antagonist,** and it acts only when aldosterone is present.

    2. **Triamterene** (*Dyrenium*) and **amiloride** (*Midamor*) act directly on the sodium–potassium transport process and are effective even after an adrenalectomy and loss of endogenous aldosterone.

    3. These drugs cause:

        a. Potassium retention

        b. Small sodium loss

        c. Weak diuresis

    4. Side effects:

        a. Hyperkalemia

            (1) The potassium-sparing diuretics are frequently combined with thiazide and loop diuretics to counteract the hypokalemia from those diuretics.

            (2) If the acute risk of cardiac arrhythmias from the hyperkalemia is high, administration of insulin will reduce the hyperkalemia by enhancing potassium uptake into cells.

        b. **Gynecomastia** can be induced by spironolactone, which is a steroid antagonist.

        c. **Menstrual irregularities** can also result from the use of spironolactone.

I. The **loop diuretics** [furosemide (*Lasix*), ethacrynic acid (*Edecrin*) and bumetanide (*Bumex*)] are so named because they act at the **thick, ascending limb of the loop of Henle.**

    1. **Sodium and chloride cotransport is blocked.**

    2. A **marked diuresis is produced,** because large amounts of sodium are reabsorbed at this site.

    3. They are effective when taken orally and are **eliminated by active proximal tubular secretion.**

        a. The secretion is important for the drugs to reach their intra-tubular site of action.

        b. Competition with the transport of uric acid at the same site can lead to hyperuricemia.

        c. They have much shorter durations of action than the thiazides.

    4. **Side effects** are more common than with the thiazides and include:

        a. Hypovolemia

        b. Hyponatremia

        c. Hypokalemia, which increases the toxicity of the cardiac glycosides

        d. Hyperuricemia

        e. Hyperglycemia

        f. Hypocalcemia, which is the opposite of the effect of the thiazides

        g. Ototoxicity, especially with ethacrynic acid. Loop diuretics should not be combined with other ototoxic drugs (e.g., aminoglycosides).

    5. The loop diuretics have a **greater diuretic efficacy than the thiazides, which have a greater efficacy than the potassium-sparing diuretics.**

J. The diuretics are useful to **mobilize edematous fluid** from many sites in the body. Important **clinical indications for administration of diuretics** include:

   1. **Congestive heart failure**—the diuretics will reduce the preload on the heart and improve heart function

   2. **Hypertension**

   3. **Hepatic ascites**

   4. **Acute pulmonary edema**

   5. **Renal failure**

   6. **Hypercalcemia**—can be treated with furosemide

   7. **Hypocalcemia**—can be treated with a thiazide

   8. **Nephrogenic diabetes insipidus**—can be treated with a thiazide

   9. **Inappropriate ADH secretion**—can be treated with furosemide and hypertonic saline

   10. **Increased intracranial pressure**—can be treated with an osmotic agent

   11. **Hyperaldosteronism**—can be treated with spironolactone

II. ANGIOTENSIN II AND ANGIOTENSIN BLOCKERS

   A. The **synthesis** of angiotensin II and III are illustrated in Figure 3–1.

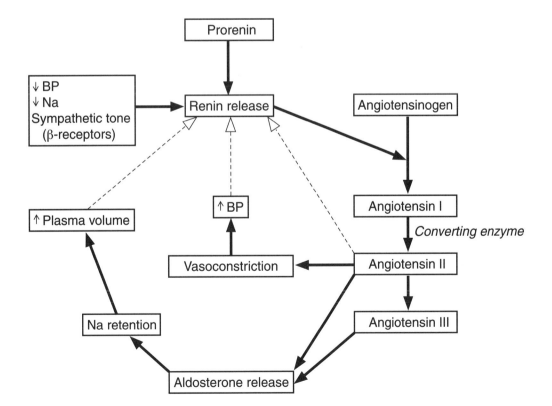

Figure 3-1. Renin-angiotensin system

   B. Effects of angiotensin II include:

     1. Vasoconstriction

     2. Increased aldosterone release

     3. Reduced renin release

   C. The primary clinical **use** of angiotensin is to **increase blood pressure.** It induces fewer cardiac arrhythmias than the catecholamines.

   D. **Angiotensin converting enzyme (ACE) can be inhibited** by several drugs.

     1. **Captopril** (*Capoten*) is an ACE inhibitor.

       a. The **effects** of ACE inhibition include:

         (1) **Reduced conversion of angiotensin I to angiotensin II**

         (2) **Reduced blood pressure**

         (3) **Reduced aldosterone levels,** which increases sodium excretion

         (4) **Increased plasma renin levels,** due to reduced feedback inhibition on renin release

         (5) **Dilation of efferent renal arterioles,** which are regulated by angiotensin II. This can reduce renal perfusion pressure.

       b. The **indications** for ACE inhibitors are:

         (1) **Hypertension**

         (2) **Congestive heart failure**

         (3) **Diabetic nephropathy**

       c. The **side effects** include:

         (1) **Hyperkalemia,** due to reduced aldosterone levels

         (2) **Hypotension**

         (3) **Coughing,** due to **increased bradykinin.** Converting enzyme also breaks down bradykinin.

         (4) **Skin rashes and angioedema**

         (3) **Fetal toxicity.** It should not be used during pregnancy.

     2. **Enalapril** (*Vasotec*) and **lisinopril** (*Prinivil,Zestril*) have the same effects as captopril, but have **longer durations of action.**

   E. The **AT1 angiotensin receptors can be inhibited by losartan** (*Cozaar*).

     1. The effects are similar to those from ACE inhibitors.

     2. **Coughing is less common** because converting enzyme is not inhibited.

III. BRADYKININ

   A. Effects

     1. A direct action on vascular smooth muscle leads to a **vasodilation.**

     2. Stimulation of the sensory nerve endings induces **pain.**

     3. Most non-vascular smooth muscle is contracted.

     4. **Capillary permeability is increased.**

   B. Bradykinin has no clinical usefulness.

IV. CALCIUM CHANNEL BLOCKERS

   A. Drugs in this class **block the slow calcium channels,** especially the voltage-sensitive L-type calcium channels. Calcium channel blockade primarily affects the cardiovascular system.

     1. Reduced calcium entry **reduces the plateau phase** (phase 2) of the action potential in the sinoatrial (SA) and atrioventricular (AV) nodes of the heart. There is little effect on the ventricular action potential, where calcium currents are less important.

2. Reduced calcium entry into vascular smooth muscle leads to a **vasodilation** and fall in blood pressure.

B. Verapamil (*Calan, Isoptin*) and **diltiazem** (*Cardizem*):

1. **Reduce heart rate**
2. **Prolong AV conduction time**
3. **Dilate coronary vessels**
4. **Dilate peripheral arterioles,** without affecting venules
5. **Reduce myocardial contractility**

C. Nifedipine (*Procardia*) a dihydropyridine, is a much **more potent arterial vasodilator** and the fall in blood pressure activates baroreceptor reflexes. As a result, the myocardial depressant effects from calcium channel blockade are counteracted, and:

1. **Heart rate is increased**
2. **AV conduction time is reduced**
3. **Myocardial contractility is increased**

D. Amlodipine (*Norvasc*) is a long-acting dihydropyridine calcium channel blocker with properties similar to nifedipine.

E. The **clinical indications** for the calcium channel blockers are:

1. **Supraventricular arrhythmias**
   a. **Paroxysmal supraventricular tachycardia (PSVT) can be acutely termi-nated.**
   b. **Atrial flutter and fibrillation are effectively treated,** because reduced AV conduction due to the calcium channel blockade reduces the ventricular rate.
2. **Angina**
3. **Hypertension**
4. **Cerebral vasospasm. Nimodipine** (*Nimotop*) has a high lipid solubility and is particularly effective.
5. **Vascular disease**
6. **Migraine headaches**

V. ANTIHYPERTENSIVES

A. Treatment with antihypertensives is usually **initiated if the blood pressure is greater than 140/90 mm Hg.** Treatment has been demonstrated to **decrease the incidence of:**

1. Stroke
2. Heart failure
3. Myocardial infarction
4. Coronary artery disease
5. Renal failure

B. **Treatment** is initiated with a **first line** drug.

1. Captopril (*Capoten*) inhibits ACE.
   a. This **reduces angiotensin synthesis** and **lowers blood pressure** by:
   (1) Vasodilating
   (2) **Reducing aldosterone release,** which increases the loss of water.
   b. There are no autonomic effects and no changes in LDL cholesterol, thus the **major side effects** are:
   (1) Hyperkalemia
   (2) Hypotension
   c. ACE inhibitors should be avoided in patients with renal artery stenosis because dilation of the efferent renal arterioles can excessively reduce the pressure in the glomerulus.

2. β-Blockers [e.g., propranolol (*Inderal*)] have many effects on blood pressure.
   a. The **mechanism** may be related to:
   (1) **Decreased heart rate and contractility**
   (2) **Decreased renin release**
   (3) **Decreased CNS sympathetic output**
   (4) **Blockade of presynaptic β-adrenoceptors** resulting in decreased norepinephrine (NE) release.
   b. The **side effects** are described in **Table 2–6.** Additional concerns are increased LDL cholesterol, increased triglycerides, and reduced high density lipoprotein (HDL) cholesterol; although these changes are small.
   c. When combined with other antihypertensives, propranolol decreases the reflex sympathetic activation of the heart and the reflex sympathetic activation of renin release.
   d. **Metoprolol is cardioselective,** thus it induces less bronchoconstriction in asthmatics and less masking of hypoglycemia in diabetics than propranolol. The β-selectivity is relative, however, and tends to disappear at high dosages.

3. Thiazide diuretics [e.g., hydrochlorothiazide (*Esidrix,HydroDIURIL*)] **initially increase sodium and water loss.**
   a. This effect is compensated for by the mechanisms illustrated in Figure 3–2.
   b. **Later,** the blood pressure is reduced as a result of a **direct vasodilation** which decreases peripheral resistance.

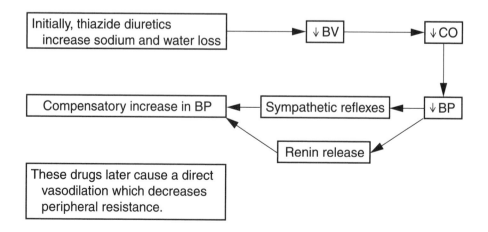

Figure 3-2. Effects of the thiazides that reduce blood pressure and activate homeostatic mechanisms

   c. **High salt intake leads to water retention which will reduce the effectiveness of the thiazides.**

   d. The **onset of the antihypertensive action is slow,** taking 2–4 weeks to develop.

   e. **Side effects** can occur, including:
   (1) Hypokalemia
      (a) To avoid hypokalemia, combine thiazide diuretics with potassium
         supplements or potassium-sparing diuretics.
      (b) This is especially important for patients on cardiac glycosides.
   (2) Hyperglycemia
   (3) **Small increases of LDL and small decreases of HDL cholesterol**

   f. The loop diuretics should be used only if the thiazides do not induce a diuresis.

4. **Calcium channel blockers** [e.g., amlodipine (*Norvasc*)] vasodilate arterioles and
   reduce blood pressure.

   a. They have no autonomic side effects and do not change the LDL cholesterol.

   b. There is an increased risk of heart attack or stroke with the short acting dihy-
   dropyridines, such as nifedipine.

C. The **second line** of drugs are the **sympathetic blockers,** which can be used alone, but
   are usually combined with a first line drug.

   1. **Prazosin** is an α_1-blocker.

   2. **Labetalol** is an α_1 and β-blocker.

   3. **Clonidine** decreases CNS sympathetic output.

   4. **Methyldopa** decreases CNS sympathetic output.

D. The **direct vasodilators** [e.g., hydralazine (*Apresoline*), minoxidil (*Loniten*)] are useful
   in combination regimens for severe hypertension.

   1. **Vasodilation of arterioles** leads to a fall in blood pressure.

   2. **Homeostatic mechanisms** (e.g., sympathetic reflexes) are induced, which com-
   pensate for the fall in blood pressure and make the arteriolar vasodilators **ineffective when used alone.** The homeostatic mechanisms include:
   a. An increase in sympathetic vasoconstrictor tone to blood vessels
   b. An increase in heart rate
   c. An increase in myocardial contractility
   d. An increase in renin release

   3. The vasodilators are usually **combined with diuretics and sympathetic blockers,**
   which will dampen the homeostatic compensatory mechanisms.

   4. **Side effects** of these drugs include:
   a. Palpitations
   b. Flushing
   c. Headache
   d. **Lupus-like syndrome with hydralazine,** especially in patients who are slow
   acetylators.
   e. **Hirsutism with minoxidil.** In fact, minoxidil is used topically (as *Rogaine*) to
   treat baldness.
   f. **Pericardial effusion with minoxidil**

VI. DRUGS FOR HYPERTENSIVE CRISES

A. Hypertensive crisis may be caused by secondary mechanisms. If it is due to **elevated
   catecholamines,** a **phentolamine test** can be used for the diagnosis.

  1. Phentolamine will **rapidly reduce blood pressure that has been elevated** due to:
   a. Pheochromocytoma
   b. Monoamine oxidase inhibitors
   c. Sympathomimetics or cocaine
   d. Clonidine withdrawal

  2. Measurement of urinary catecholamine metabolites is also diagnostic.

  3. Treatment of hypertensive crises due to elevated catecholamines involves the administration of:
   a. α- and β-blockers
   b. Labetalol
   c. Metyrosine, an inhibitor of tyrosine hydroxylase

B. Hypertensive crises due to other causes will not respond so dramatically to phentolamine and are treated with rapid-acting antihypertensives, usually administered i.v.

  1. Sodium nitroprusside (*Nitropress*), like the nitrates, **dilates venules** and **arterioles.**
   a. The onset of action is **very rapid,** within minutes.
   b. The half-life is **very short,** which makes the antihypertensive effect **very controllable,** but it requires regular monitoring.
   c. Side effects include:
    (1) Hypotension
    (2) Toxicity from thiocyanate and cyanide, which are by-products of nitroprusside metabolism.

  2. Fenoldopam (*Corlopam*), is a **D_1-dopamine receptor agonist** that
   a. dilates peripheral arterioles, especially **renal and mesenteric arterioles**
   b. Has a **rapid onset** after i.v. infusion
   c. Has a **very short half-life**

  3. Nitroglycerin, i.v. has actions similar to nitroprussido, although the venous dilation is more pronounced than the arterial dilation.

  4. Diazoxide (*Hyperstat I.V.*), like hydralazine, **dilates only arterioles.**
   a. Side effects include:
    (1) Palpitations
    (2) Hyperglycemia
   b. It can **aggravate angina.**

  5. Labetalol (*Normodyne, Trandate*), when administered intravenously, has a rapid antihypertensive action.

VII. DRUGS FOR ANGINA PECTORIS

A. Patients with angina (stable, variant, or unstable types) develop **S-T segment elevation or depression** on the electrocardiogram (EKG) during myocardial hypoxia. This can be induced diagnostically by:

  1. Treadmill stress testing

  2. Ergonovine, which induces a coronary vasoconstriction

  3. Dobutamine, which increases heart rate and contractility

B. Treatment of angina is oriented to reducing oxygen demand or increasing oxygen supply to the heart.

  1. Nitrates, which are useful for all types of angina, act directly on vascular smooth muscle cells.
   a. They dilate vessels in a manner similar to nitric oxide. Endothelium-derived relaxing factor (EDRF) is probably nitric oxide.

   (1) The primary effect is a **reduction in venous tone,** which leads to venous pooling and reduced venous return (reduced preload).
   (2) Arteriolar tone is less effectively reduced, and leads to reduced peripheral resistance (reduced afterload) and reduced blood pressure.
   (3) Both effects reduce the myocardial wall stress and thereby **reduce the oxygen consumption** of the heart.
   (4) Dilation of collateral coronary vessels and coronary vessels in spasm are additional minor effects.
   b. Short and long acting **preparations** are available.
   (1) **Nitroglycerin** (*Nitrostat*) is administered **sublingually** to terminate an acute anginal attack.
      (a) The onset is very rapid and the half–life is short (1–3 minutes).
      (b) Oral administration is ineffective for the treatment of an acute attack due to a high first–pass metabolism.
   (2) High doses of nitroglycerin (*Nitro-Bid*), which saturate the metabolic enzymes, can be administered orally or topically for prophylaxis.
   (3) **Isosorbide dinitrate** (*Isordil*) is a long-acting nitrate that is also useful for prophylaxis.
   c. **Side effects** from the nitrates include:
   (1) **Headache** from the vascular dilation
   (2) **Syncope** from the **postural hypotension**
   (3) **Reflex tachycardia,** which may occasionally induce an anginal attack
   (4) **Methemoglobinemia,** which can be reversed by methylene blue
   (5) **Tolerance and withdrawal symptoms,** such as anginal attacks during withdrawal from high-dose, long-term therapy

2. **β-Blockers** produce several beneficial effects.
   a. β-Blockade of the heart is the primary mode of action.
   (1) Exercise-induced tachycardia and exercise-induced increases in myocardial contractility are reduced.
   (2) Blood pressure is decreased (decreased afterload).
   (3) Heart rate is reduced, which increases endocardial perfusion time.
   (4) Reflex tachycardia from the nitrates is reduced, making the combination of nitrates and β-blockers quite useful.
   b. **Propranolol should be avoided** or used with caution in patients with:
   (1) **Variant angina,** as blockade of β-adrenoceptors (dilatory) in the coronary vessels may increase the coronary spasm
   (2) **Asthma,** due to a bronchoconstricting effect
   (3) **Congestive heart failure,** due to the depressant effect on myocardial contractility
   (4) **Calcium channel blockers,** as both classes of drugs depress myocardial contractility
   c. **Propranolol is used prophylactically for 1.5 to 3 years after an acute MI to decrease the ischemic damage.**
   d. The side effects of β-blockers have been previously described (See Table 2–6). It is important to **avoid rapid withdrawal** from treatment, which can induce anginal attacks.

3. **Calcium channel blockers** [e.g., verapamil (*Calan, Isoptin*)] are effective for the treatment of all types of angina, and may be used in combination with the nitrates or the β-blockers or both. Calcium channel blockers
   a. Decrease heart rate
   b. Decrease myocardial contractility

    c. **Vasodilate arterioles** (decrease afterload)

    d. **Dilate coronary vessels,** which reduces coronary spasm

VIII. CARDIAC GLYCOSIDES

A. **Mild chronic congestive heart failure can be treated with** drugs that reduce the preload and/or afterload on the heart, such as

    1. **ACE inhibitors,** which are the drugs of choice

    2. **β-blocker,** e.g. carvedilol, to block sympathetic effects on the heart and vasculature

    3. **Diuretics,** e.g. spironolactone, to block the effects of aldosterone

    4. **α_1-Blocker,** e.g. prazosin, to block sympathetic effects on the vasculature.

B. More severe heart failure often requires the administration of the cardiac glycosides which are derived from the foxglove (*Digitalis*) plant.

C. The **glycosides inhibit Na^+/K^+ ATPase,** which **reduces active Na^+/K^+ transport** and increases the intracellular concentrations of sodium and **calcium** ions. The elevated free calcium ion concentration enhances myocardial contractility.

    1. The effect on ventricular performance is shown in Figure 3–3.
        a. No net change of oxygen consumption occurs.
        b. The efficiency of myocardial contractions is improved.

    2. The increased contractility leads to a cascade of events shown in Figure 3–4.

D. Two glycosides are used clinically.

    1. **Digoxin** (*Lanoxin*) has a bioavailability of 75% and a volume of distribution (V_d) of 6 l/kg, due to accumulation in tissues, but not in fat. Generic preparations are not reliably bioequivalent.
        a. It is **eliminated primarily by glomerular filtration in the kidney,** thus the **creatinine clearance** is useful in determining the maintenance dose.
        b. The **half-life is 36 hours,** which means that a steady state serum drug concentration is not achieved for 6–8 days (without a loading dose).
        c. For a rapid onset of action, use a divided loading dose to avoid toxicity.

    2. **Digitoxin** (*Crystodigin*) is more lipid soluble and has a bioavailability of 100%.
        a. It is 97% bound to plasma proteins.

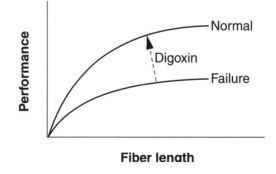

Figure 3-3. Effect of digoxin on myocardial contractility.

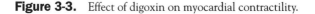

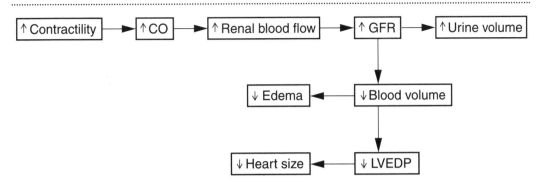

Figure 3-4. Effects resulting from the increase in myocardial contractility induced by digoxin. CO=cardiac output; *GFR*=glomerular filtration rate; *LVEDP*=left ventricular end-diastolic pressure

      b. Digitoxin is **cleared by metabolism** in the liver and the metabolite is eliminated in the bile. 25% is reabsorbed (enterohepatic cycling).

      c. The **half-life is 5–7 days.**

  E. The **indications** for the glycosides are:

    1. **Severe, chronic congestive heart failure,** but not high output, obstructive, or pulmonary failure (**Hypertrophic cardiomyopathy,** which can lead to heart failure, is best treated with **β-blockers** or **calcium channel blockers** to reduce heart rate and thereby enhance the filling of the heart.)

    2. **Supraventricular arrhythmias** (e.g., atrial flutter and atrial fibrillation). The glycosides reduce the ventricular rate by inducing partial AV nodal block.

  F. **Side effects** are very common, because there is considerable overlap between the therapeutic and toxic serum concentration ranges.

    1. **Cardiac toxicities** can be life-threatening.

      a. **Vagal enhancement** can lead to **bradycardia** and **AV nodal block** (indirect effects). These side effects can be treated with atropine.

      b. **Direct actions** on the myocardium (from ATPase inhibition) can lead to **arrhythmias** that are accentuated by hypokalemia (e.g., from diuretics). This side effect can be treated with potassium or lidocaine.

    2. **Non-cardiac** effects are usually not life-threatening.

      a. **Nausea and vomiting** occurs due to activation of the chemoreceptor trigger zone (CTZ) in the CNS.

      b. Enhanced vagal activity can lead to **diarrhea.**

      c. **Color vision** can be distorted.

  G. If the toxicity is mild (and serum potassium is in the normal range), withdraw the glycoside and restart at a lower dose. If toxicity is life-threatening, administer digoxin immune F_{ab} (*Digibind*).

  H. **Drug interactions** are common.

    1. **Hypokalemia** or **hypercalcemia** increase toxicity.

    2. Reduced renal clearance of digoxin, leading to increased toxicity, occurs with:

      a. Quinidine

      b. **Calcium channel blockers**

      c. **Hypothyroidism**

IX. ANTIARRHYTHMICS

A. There are 5 phases in the cardiac action potential:

1. Phase 0—upstroke due to the sodium current

2. Phase 1—peak

3. Phase 2—plateau due to the calcium current

4. Phase 3—repolarization due to the potassium current

5. Phase 4—diastolic depolarization

B. **Bradyarrhythmias** can be treated with **atropine or β-agonists.**

C. **Tachyarrhythmias** can be treated with the **antiarrhythmics,** which depress the electrical activity of the myocardial cells. The antiarrhythmics reduce tachyarrhythmias by:

1. **Decreasing ectopic automaticity**

2. **Enhancing or depressing conduction,** to reduce reentry

D. There are **4 primary mechanisms** of **antiarrhythmic action,** including:

1. Sodium channel blockade

2. β-Blockade

3. Increased refractoriness

4. Calcium channel blockade

E. Class IA antiarrhythmics are **sodium channel blockers** (direct action) with anticholinergic activity (indirect action).

1. The **effects** of the two actions are illustrated in **Table 3–1.**

2. The changes of the myocardial action potential are illustrated in Figure 3–5.

a. The **slowing of the diastolic depolarization** (Phase 4) leads to the reduced automaticity.

b. The **slowing of the rate of rise** of the action potential (Phase O) leads to the reduced excitability and reduced conduction velocity.

c. The **prolongation** of the action potential leads to the increased effective refractory period.

3. The **indirect actions** from the **anticholinergic activity** only occur at the SA and AV nodes because these are the primary sites of parasympathetic innervation.

Table 3-1
Changes in Myocardial Cell Properties due to the Direct (Sodium Channel Block) and Indirect (Vagal Block) Actions of the Group IA Antiarrhythmics

Sodium channel block	Vagal block (SA and AV nodes)
↓ automaticity	↑ automaticity
↓ excitability	↑ excitability
↑ effective refractory period	↓ effective refractory period

Sum total of effects of IA antiarrhythmics:
   SA and AV nodes—variable effects
   atrial and ventricular muscle—direct effects	

AV=atrioventricular; SA=sinoatrial; ↑=increased; ↓=decreased

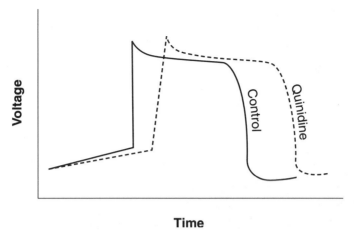

Figure 3-5. Changes in the myocardial action potential induced by Class IA antiarrhythmics (e.g., quinidine)

   a. The net effect of the IA antiarrhythmics at the SA and AV nodes is variable, depending upon whether the direct or indirect effects predominate.
   b. At atrial and ventricular muscle, the direct effects predominate, because there is little parasympathetic innervation.

4. Class IA antiarrhythmics are **often combined with the cardiac glycosides.**
   a. The indirect effects (anticholinergic) of the antiarrhythmic oppose the indirect effects (vagomimetic) of the cardiac glycoside.
   b. The combination results in little indirect activity, and leads to sodium channel blockade with increased myocardial contractility.

5. Several Class IA antiarrhythmics are commonly used.
   a. **Quinidine** (*Quinidex,Cardioquin*) is only used orally, as parenteral administration has marked hypotensive effects.
      (1) The side effects include **cinchonism,** which is characterized by ringing in the ears, blurred vision, nausea, and vomiting.
      (2) **Thrombocytopenia** can also be induced.
      (3) Quinidine reduces the renal elimination of digoxin, which can lead to an increase in the toxicity from digoxin.
   b. **Procainamide** (*Pronestyl*) can be used orally or intravenously.
      (1) N-Acetylprocainamide is an active metabolite.
      (2) **A lupus-like syndrome** can be induced, especially in those patients who have a **slow acetylator phenotype.**
   c. **Disopyramide** (*Norpace*) is an oral antiarrhythmic that is also the most potent antimuscarinic.

6. Some **side effects** are common to all Class IA antiarrhythmics.
   a. **Ventricular arrhythmias** induced by the Class IA antiarrhythmics can lead to **syncope.**
   b. **AV block** induced by the Class IA antiarrhythmics can lead to an **increased P-R interval.**
   c. There may also be increased QRS and QT intervals. The polymorphic ven-

tricular arrhythmia, *torsades de pointes*, can be induced by the prolonged QT interval.

   d. **Decreased contractility** can aggravate heart failure, especially with disopyramide.

   e. A direct **vasodilation** can lower blood pressure.

7. Uses for Class IA antiarrhythmic drugs are:

   a. **Treatment and prophylactic control of symptomatic ventricular tachyarrhythmias**

   b. **Prophylactic control of supraventricular arrhythmias.**

F. **Class IB** antiarrhythmic drugs are **sodium channel blockers** without anticholinergic activity.

   1. Lidocaine (*Xylocaine*) is a very effective **parenteral** antiarrhythmic.

   a. It is rapidly metabolized in the liver **(high extraction ratio)** and has a low bioavailability (0.3); thus it is not used orally.

   (1) **Heart failure** will decrease the liver blood flow and thereby slow the metabolism of lidocaine.

   (2) The **maintenance dose** of lidocaine should be **reduced** in patients with heart failure.

   b. The **elimination of lidocaine** follows **2 compartment** kinetics (Figure 3–6), thus repeated dosing will increase the duration of the therapeutic effect.

   c. The **effects** of lidocaine **on the myocardial action potential** are illustrated in **Figure 3–7.**

   (1) **Automaticity is decreased.**

   (2) **Excitability is decreased.**

   (3) **The effective refractory period is decreased,** which is unexpected.

   d. The actions of lidocaine on myocardial muscle are **frequency-dependent,** with the highest activity at the higher frequencies. Thus it acts preferentially on arrhythmic muscle.

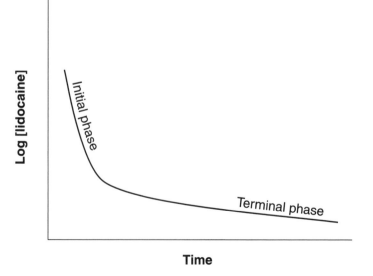

Figure 3-6. Lidocaine concentration versus time relationship, which displays two phases (two compartments)

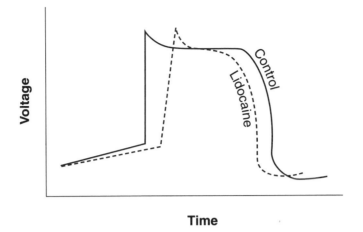

Figure 3-7. Changes in the myocardial action potential induced by Class IB antiarrhythmics (e.g., lidocaine)

    e. There are **few side effects,** however **at large dosages** it can:
        (1) Produce local anesthetic side effects, such as **tremors** and **convulsions**
        (2) **Reduce myocardial contractility**
        (3) Slow AV conduction
    f. The **indications** for the use of lidocaine are limited to **ventricular** tachyarrhythmias, including:
        (1) Ventricular tachycardia
        (2) **Premature ventricular complexes**
        (3) **Ventricular fibrillation**
        (4) **Digitalis-induced ventricular arrhythmias**

2. **Mexiletine** (*Mexitil*) has effects that are similar to lidocaine, however
    a. It is **effective when given orally,** as there is no first–pass metabolism.
    b. The half-life is much **longer.**

3. **Phenytoin** (*Dilantin*), an anticonvulsant, also has antiarrhythmic effects.

G. **Class IC** antiarrhythmic drugs [e.g., **flecainide** (*Tambocor*)] induce marked reductions of the sodium permeability changes.

H. **Class II** antiarrhythmics are the **β-blockers** [e.g., propranolol (*Inderal*)].

    1. They act primarily by **reducing the effects of the sympathetic nervous system on the myocardium.**
        a. **Phase 4 depolarization is reduced,** leading to a reduction of automaticity and conduction velocity in the SA node, AV node and Purkinje fibers.
        b. **Excitability is reduced.**
        c. The effective refractory period of the AV node is increased.

    2. High doses may induce sodium channel blockade.

    3. Indications for β-blockers include:
        a. **Sympathetic-induced tachyarrhythmias**
        b. **PSVT** (because β-blockers reduce reentry at the AV node)
        c. **Atrial flutter and fibrillation** (because β-blockers slow AV conduction, thereby reducing the ventricular rate)
        d. **Prophylaxis after an acute MI** (because β-blockers reduce sudden death)

I. Class III antiarrhythmics **prolong the action potential and the effective refractory period.**

    1. Amiodarone (*Cordarone*) increases the refractory period.

        a. It **acts at all sites** in the myocardium, which is unusual for an antiarrhythmic, and it effectively reduces almost any arrhythmia.

        b. The **half-life is very long,** approximately 30 days.

        c. **Toxicity is very high,** including:

            (1) **Pneumonitis.** Pulmonary toxicity is fatal in 10% of patients affected.

            (2) Change of thyroid function

    2. Bretylium (*Bretylol*) decreases catecholamine release, prolongs the action potential, and increases the effective refractory period in the myocardium.

    3. Sotalol (*Betapace*) is a non-selective β-blocker with Class III activity.

    4. Ibutilide (*Corvert*), given i.v. prolongs the action potential and can be used to **convert atrial flutter or fibrillation to normal sinus rhythm.**

J. Class IV antiarrhythmics are the **calcium channel blockers** [e.g., **verapamil** (*Calan, Isoptin*)].

    1. Calcium channels are particularly important for action potential generation in the SA and AV nodes.

    2. Blockade of the L-type calcium channels **decreases heart rate, slows AV conduction,** and **increases the effective refractory period.**

    3. Verapamil has a low bioavailability (F = 0.2), due to first-pass metabolism, and 80%–90% of the verapamil in the serum is bound to plasma proteins.

    4. **Indications** for the calcium channel blockers include supraventricular arrhythmias, such as:

        a. **PSVT**

        b. **Atrial flutter**

        c. **Atrial fibrillation**

    5. **Side effects** of verapamil include:

        a. **Bradycardia**

        b. **AV block**

        c. **Excessive ventricular rate in patients with Wolff-Parkinson-White syndrome who are being treated for atrial fibrillation**

        d. **Heart failure,** due to reduced myocardial contractility

        e. Constipation

    6. The effects of the calcium channel blockers on the myocardium can be antagonized by the catecholamines, digoxin, or calcium.

K. **Miscellaneous** antiarrhythmics are also useful.

    1. **Adenosine** (*Adenocard*) hyperpolarizes supraventricular muscle membranes, and it is used to **terminate PSVT.** The duration of action is only one minute.

    2. **Digoxin** (*Lanoxin*) has antiarrhythmic effects, due to a **depression of AV nodal conduction.**

        a. Increased myocardial contractility and the long duration of action of digoxin are unusual for antiarrhythmics.

        b. Uses include:

            (1) **Atrial flutter and fibrillation**

            (2) **PSVT**

            (3) **Arrhythmias in patients with congestive heart failure**

3. **Phenylephrine** increases blood pressure, which reflexly reduces heart rate and reduces PSVT.

X. ANTICOAGULANTS

A. Heparin (*Liquaemin*) is an **acidic mucopolysaccharide.**

   1. High endogenous concentrations occur in the mast cells in the lungs.

   2. It is a **very large, polar,** and **water-soluble molecule.**
   a. It must be **given intravenously** or **subcutaneously.**
   b. Distribution is limited to the **vascular space.**
   c. **Inactivation** is due to **metabolism,** which follows **zero–order kinetics.** Increasing the dose increases the time to eliminate 50% of the drug.

   3. It acts by **catalyzing** the reaction between **antithrombin III** and **thrombin,** which results in an inactive complex of thrombin.
   a. It also **complexes factor Xa.**
   b. The onset of action is **immediate.**
   c. The goal of treatment is to increase the **activated partial thromboplastin time (APTT)** by approximately **2 times** the normal value.

   4. **Side effects** include:
   a. **Hemorrhage**
   b. **Thrombocytopenia,** which is immunologically mediated.

   5. **Protamine,** a basic compound which **complexes heparin,** is the **antidote** for heparin.

   6. **Low molecular weight heparins, e.g. enoxaparin** (*Lovenox*):
   a. **Act only on factor Xa.** Monitor the Xa concentration rather than APTT.
   b. Are better absorbed after subcutaneous injection than heparin
   c. Are eliminated by the kidney, by **first order kinetics.** They should not be used in patients with renal failure.
   d. Have a more predictable dose-response relationship than heparin
   e. Have a lower incidence of thrombocytopenia than heparin

B. Warfarin (*Coumadin,Panwarfin*) is an **oral anticoagulant.**

   1. Blockade of the reduction of vitamin K to its active form slows the carboxylation and **decreases the synthesis of vitamin K-dependent clotting factors** (II, VII, IX and X).
   a. The **onset of action is delayed** (8–12 hours), because stores of the clotting factors must be depleted.
   b. The maximum anticoagulant effect of warfarin occurs after 1 week of administration.
   c. The therapeutic goal is an INR (International Normalized Ratio) of 2 to 3, which will approximately double the prothrombin time.

   2. Because warfarin is **effective when given orally,** it is more useful than heparin for outpatients.

   3. **Many drug interactions** can occur.
   a. Extensive plasma protein binding (99%) can result in competition with other drugs for the binding sites.
   b. Metabolism of warfarin in the liver can be enhanced by many other drugs.

   4. The **side effects** include:
   a. **Hemorrhage,** which can be reversed by the **antidotes, vitamin K or vitamin-K dependent clotting factors.**

    b. Skin necrosis, due to thrombosis of the microvasculature in the skin.

    c. Teratogenicity, because it readily crosses the placenta and affects the developing fetus.

  5. Acute anticoagulant therapy is often initiated with both heparin and warfarin. As the warfarin becomes effective, the heparin is withdrawn.

  6. Warfarin and heparin slow the production of a clot, but they do not dissolve clots.

C. Fibrinolytics dissolve clots.

  1. **Tissue plasminogen activator (tPA, alteplase), urokinase, streptokinase** and **anistreplase** enhance the formation of plasmin from plasminogen.

    a. The plasmin breaks down fibrin, thereby dissolving clots.

    b. Dissolution of clots by **intracoronary administration of a fibrinolytic** can restore coronary blood flow after an **MI.**

      (1) This will reduce myocardial damage, if given within a few hours of the MI.

      (2) It can also induce hemorrhaging at other sites.

    c. Dissolution of clots in the brain by fibrinolytics can reduce the CNS injury after a **thrombotic stroke.** It must not be used after a hemorrhagic stroke.

  2. The **antidote** for the fibrinolytics is **aminocaproic acid,** a plasmin antagonist.

D. Antiplatelet drugs, given prophylactically, reduce the incidence of MI and stroke.

  1. **Low doses of aspirin inhibit cyclooxygenase** which **decreases thromboxane synthesis,** thereby decreasing platelet aggregation.

  2. Dipyridamole (*Persantine*) decreases platelet adhesiveness.

XI. DRUGS FOR SHOCK

A. The treatment for each type of shock will be quite different.

B. **Avoid vasoconstrictors** if the sympathetic nervous system has already compromised blood flow to the peripheral tissues.

C. **Use fluids, vasodilators, and inotropic drugs.** Dopamine is particularly useful because it will dilate the renal and mesenteric vasculature.

XII. ANTIHYPERLIPIDEMICS

A. The first mode of therapy for hypercholesterolemias is **modification of the diet** to reduce fat and caloric intake.

B. Lovastatin (*Mevacor*) **simvastatin** (*Zocor*) and **atorvastatin** (*Lipitor*) **competitively inhibit hydroxymethylglutarylCoA** (HMG CoA) **reductase.**

  1. This enzyme is the **rate limiting** step in the synthesis of cholesterol.

  2. Reduced cholesterol synthesis leads to an increase in the number of hepatic **LDL receptors,** which enhance the uptake of LDL cholesterol from the serum.

    a. **Serum LDL cholesterol is reduced.**

    b. HDL cholesterol is slightly increased.

    c. Triglycerides are slightly reduced.

    d. The risk of MI is reduced.

  3. **Side effects** from lovastatin include

    a. **Hepatotoxicity**

    b. Myositis, an inflammation of skeletal muscle.

C. Cholestyramine (*Questran*) and **colestipol** (*Colestid*) are **quaternary ammonium ion-exchange resins** that are **not absorbed** from the intestine.

  1. They **bind bile salts** and eliminate them in the feces.
     a. Bile salt synthesis from cholesterol is increased.
     b. Cholesterol content in the liver is reduced.
     c. The liver increases the number of LDL receptors, which lowers the serum LDL cholesterol.

  2. Side effects include:
     a. Abdominal discomfort and constipation.
     b. Binding of fat-soluble vitamins and anionic drugs
     c. An increase in very low density lipoproteins (VLDL) and triglycerides.

D. Niacin (nicotinic acid, vitamin B_3) at high dosages has antihyperlipidemic actions.

  1. Many effects occur and the exact mechanism is unclear.
     a. It decreases lipolysis in adipose tissue which decreases the free fatty acids in the plasma.
     b. Triglyceride synthesis is markedly reduced, which decreases the hepatic secretion of VLDL.
     c. Decreased LDL production leads to reduced serum cholesterol.

  2. A common **side effect** is **cutaneous flushing,** due to **prostaglandin** release. This effect can be reduced by inhibiting prostaglandin synthesis with **aspirin.**

E. Gemfibrozil (*Lopid*) and **clofibrate** (*Atromid-S*) are more active in **lowering triglycerides.**

  1. **Increases in lipoprotein lipase activity** lead to a reduction of VLDL, which predominantly transports triglycerides.

  2. Elimination of cholesterol in the bile is also enhanced which can lead to **gallstones** as a **side effect.**

4

Central Neuropharmacology

I. PRINCIPLES OF GENERAL ANESTHESIA

A. The **primary objectives** of general anesthesia are:

1. Amnesia

2. Analgesia

3. Blunting of consciousness

4. Suppression of autonomic reflexes

5. Muscle relaxation

B. Due to the blood-brain barrier, all central nervous system (CNS) drugs including the general anesthetics must either be **lipid soluble** or carried across the barrier by active transport, e.g., P-glycoproteins, in order to be effective.

C. The mechanism of action of general anesthetics has been difficult to determine.

1. Classical theories involve a **physical association** of anesthetics with cell membranes. This leads to several implications.

a. The **potency** of each gaseous anesthetic, characterized by the **minimal anesthetic concentration (MAC),** is directly related to the **oil-water partition coefficient** for that anesthetic.

b. The association of the anesthetic with cell membranes **reduces the excitability** of the membranes.

c. There are **no receptors** for the inhalation anesthetics.

d. There are **no specific antagonists** for the inhalation anesthetics.

2. Recent theories involve an **enhancement of the effects of inhibitory neurotransmitters, e.g., GABA.**

D. At low concentrations of a general anesthetic the CNS is depressed more than other tissues; but as the concentration is increased, all excitable cells are eventually depressed.

E. Anesthetics induce characteristic stages of anesthesia. These were first described for anesthesia with diethyl ether, but occur with other anesthetics as well.

1. Stage 1 involves **analgesia.**

2. Stage 2 involves **excitement,** due to **blockade of inhibitory pathways** in the brain. This can be a dangerous phase, due to the vomiting, restlessness, and other hyperexcitable effects that may occur.

3. **Stage 3** is the stage at which **surgery is usually performed,** and Stage 3 is divided into four planes.

4. **Stage 4** involves **respiratory and cardiovascular depression,** which, if pronounced, can lead to death.

F. The inhalation anesthetics act as gases in the body and follow the **gas laws.**

1. **Dalton's Law.** An anesthetic exerts a partial pressure that is proportional to the percent of the anesthetic in the mixture.

2. **Fick's Law.** The anesthetic diffuses down its concentration gradient.

3. **Henry's Law.** The amount of anesthetic dissolved in a liquid is proportional to the partial pressure of the anesthetic in the mixture.

G. The **rate of induction** of anesthesia is **dependent on the blood solubility of an anesthetic.**

1. The blood solubility can be determined by measuring the blood–gas partition coefficient (λ).

2. High blood solubility leads to a slow rise in the partial pressure of the anesthetic in the body and a slow induction.

3. The induction of highly blood soluble anesthetics is most readily hastened by hyperventilation.

H. The factors affecting distribution vary with the phase.

1. The **initial distribution** of an anesthetic will be dependent on the relative **tissue blood flows,** and more anesthetic will go to areas with the higher blood flows.

2. The **final distribution** will be dependent on the **tissue-blood partition coefficients,** although the tissue-blood partition coefficients for most anesthetics in most tissues is approximately one.
   a. An exception is the fat-blood partition coefficient which is usually high (25–60).
   b. Movement of an anesthetic into fat will be slow due to the low blood supply to fat. Only after long anesthesias will significant amounts of anesthetic be sequestered in fat.
   c. Recovery from long anesthesias may be slower than anticipated due to the slow elimination of anesthetic from fat.

II. INHALATION ANESTHETICS

A. **Diethyl ether** was the first useful anesthetic.

1. It has several major disadvantages, including:
   a. **Very slow induction** ($\lambda = 16$)
   b. **Flammability**
   c. **Respiratory irritation,** which frequently leads to enhanced secretions, nausea and vomiting

2. It is, however, a complete anesthetic, meaning that it:
   a. Induces muscle relaxation, due to actions on the spinal cord and neuromuscular junction
   b. Induces analgesia
   c. Induces unconsciousness
   d. Maintains respiration and circulation

B. As compared to diethyl ether, the newer inhalation anesthetics, which are **halogenated hydrocarbons,** are

1. Less soluble in blood, resulting in **faster rates of induction and recovery**

2. Non-flammable

3. **Less irritating** to the respiratory tract

C. The newer anesthetics do have some common **disadvantages,** in that they

1. **Depress respiration**

2. **Decrease blood pressure** in a dose-related fashion

3. Dilate cerebral blood vessels which can increase intracranial pressure

4. Relax the uterus during pregnancy

5. Induce a low incidence of malignant hyperthermia, which can be treated with dantrolene

6. Have weaker analgesic actions

D. Specific properties of the halogenated hydrocarbon inhalation anesthetics are shown in Table 4-1.

1. Halothane (*Fluothane*) was the first anesthetic in this group.
   a. It is a **poor skeletal muscle relaxant and a poor analgesic,** thus it is usually combined with other drugs (e.g., muscle relaxants and analgesics). The combination is called balanced anesthesia.
   b. Halothane **sensitizes the myocardium to catecholamines,** thus arrhythmias may occur when catecholamines are administered.
   c. **Metabolism of halothane** to halogenated products is high, which may account for the infrequent **hepatotoxicity.**

2. Enflurane (*Ethrane*) can induce **seizure patterns** during anesthesia.

3. Isoflurane (*Forane*) has **respiratory irritant** effects.

4. Sevoflurane (*Ultane*) is partially metabolized by the liver.

5. Desflurane (*Suprane*) has the **fastest** onset of and recovery from anesthesia. It also has **respiratory irritant** effects.

E. **Nitrous oxide** is a gas with:

1. A rapid onset and recovery ($\lambda = 0.4$)

2. **Excellent analgesic activity**

Table 4-1
Properties of Halogenated Inhalation Anesthetics

	Halothane	**Enflurane**	**Isoflurane**	**Sevoflurane**	**Desflurane**
Induction speed (λ)	2.3	1.8	1.4	0.7	0.4
Irritation of respiratory tract	low	low	moderate	low	moderate
Muscle relaxation	low	moderate	moderate	moderate	moderate
Myocardial depression	high	moderate	low	high	low
Sensitization of myocardium	high	moderate	low	low	low
% Metabolized	20	2	0.2	3	0.02

3. No effect on the function of most vital systems

4. **Inadequate potency,** leading to:
   a. Unconsciousness only when used with other anesthetics
   b. **A second gas effect** during induction which accelerates the onset of anesthesia by other inhalation anesthetics
   c. **Diffusion hypoxia** during recovery, due to the filling of the lungs with nitrous oxide so that inadequate oxygen is inhaled. This can be avoided by administering **100% oxygen** for a short time at the conclusion of the nitrous oxide anesthesia.

F. Several **miscellaneous** anesthetics are of historical interest.

   1. **Methoxyflurane** is:
      a. **The most potent anesthetic** available for clinical use
      b. **The best analgesic** anesthetic
      c. **Nephrotoxic** and thus seldom used

   2. **Cyclopropane** is an explosive gas.

   3. **Chloroform** is:
      a. A complete anesthetic
      b. Hepatotoxic

III. INTRAVENOUS ANESTHETICS

A. **Barbiturates,** such as **thiopental** (*Pentothal*) have a rapid onset of anesthesia due to a **high lipid solubility.**

   1. When administered it goes primarily to areas of high blood flow, such as the brain.

   2. The short duration of anesthesia is due to **redistribution** from the brain to peripheral tissues with lower blood flows, such as skeletal muscle.

   3. Clearance from the body by metabolism is very slow.

   4. The duration of anesthesia becomes longer with repeated administrations because less redistribution can occur. As a result, the primary **uses** of thiopental are for:
      a. **Induction** of anesthesia
      b. **Short anesthesias**

   5. The anesthetic has the following **properties:**
      a. **Marked respiratory and cardiovascular depression,** especially with a rapid bolus injection
      b. Weak skeletal muscle relaxant activity
      c. **Antianalgesic** activity (increases sensitivity to pain)
      d. Pharyngeal stimulation
      e. **Very alkaline** solution, which creates problems if improperly administered

B. **Propofol** (*Diprivan*) also has a rapid onset of action and recovery.

   1. Although the anesthesia is terminated by redistribution, there are **no cumulative effects** and it can be used for long anesthesias.

   2. The **postoperative complications (e.g., nausea, vomiting, residual drowsiness) are less than with other i.v. anesthetics.**

   3. It can markedly reduce blood pressure.

C. **Opioids,** such as **fentanyl** (*Sublimaze*), **sufentanil** (*Sufenta*) and **alfentanil** (*Alfenta*), are potent **narcotic analgesics.**

   1. They have the following anesthetic properties:

  a. Good analgesia

  b. Euphoria

  c. Respiratory depression, which can be reversed by naloxone

  d. Muscle rigidity

  e. Nausea and vomiting

 2. The anesthesia is very safe with little cardiovascular depression.

 3. **Droperidol** (*Inapsine*), an **antipsychotic** or neuroleptic, can be combined with fentanyl (*Innovar*) to induce neuroleptanalgesia.

  a. The patient is conscious and can respond.

  b. It can be supplemented with nitrous oxide to induce unconsciousness (neuroleptanesthesia).

D. **Midazolam** (*Versed*) is a **water soluble benzodiazepine** with a rapid onset of action and a short duration.

 1. The patient remains conscious at low doses, but experiences amnesia during the anesthesia.

 2. At high doses some loss of consciousness is induced.

 3. It can induce respiratory depression that is reversible by administration of benzodiazepine antagonists, such as flumazenil (*Romazicon*).

E. **Ketamine** (*Ketalar*) is an analogue of phencyclidine, a hallucinogen.

 1. It induces a **dissociative anesthesia.**

  a. The patient is awake

  b. The analgesic effects are excellent

  c. Muscle tone is either unchanged or increased.

  d. Blood pressure is often increased.

  e. Respiration is not affected.

 2. Ketamine can be administered intravenously or intramuscularly.

 3. **Side effects** are related to hallucinogenic activity, which leads to:

  a. **Vivid dreams**

  b. **Hallucinations,** which can be reduced by diazepam

IV. LOCAL ANESTHETICS

A. **A reduction of the changes of the** P_{Na} **and** P_K in the activated nerve membrane leads to local anesthesia.

 1. There are no effects on the resting membrane.

 2. The effects on the nerve action potential of both sensory and motor nerve fibers include:

  a. A reduction in the amplitude

  b. A reduction in the rate of rise

  c. A reduction in conduction velocity

  d. A blockade of axonal conduction

 3. Sensory neurons are blocked before motor neurons because the sensory axons are usually smaller and have less myelin.

B. Local anesthetics have 3 common **structural components,** except for benzocaine (Figure 4–1).

 1. The **aromatic** residue is **lipophilic,** which is important for good membrane penetration.

Lidocaine

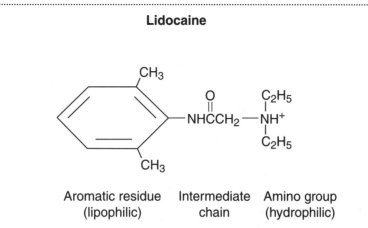

Aromatic residue   Intermediate   Amino group
(lipophilic)   chain   (hydrophilic)

Figure 4-1. General structure of local anesthetics, as illustrated by the amide, lidocaine.

2. The **amino** group is **hydrophilic.**
   a. It can become charged by picking up a proton.
   b. pH and pK_a determine whether the local anesthetic is present predominantly in the charged or uncharged forms.
      (1) Only the uncharged form crosses the nerve cell membrane (Figure 4–2).
      (2) It is converted to the **charged form** inside the axon, which then interacts with binding sites within the ion channels.
      (3) Stock solutions of local anesthetics are acidic (local anesthetic is ionized). The acidity must be neutralized before anesthesia can occur.
      (4) Local anesthetics will be less effective for inducing anesthesia in areas of inflammation because:
         (a) The pH is low
         (b) Most of the anesthetic will be charged and unable to penetrate the nerve cell membrane
      (5) Mucous membranes have a low buffering capacity and cannot readily neutralize the acidity of the local anesthetic solution. As a result, mucous membranes are relatively difficult to anesthetize.
   c. The pK_a must be between 7 and 9 so that some of the local anesthetic is present in the charged form and some is present in the uncharged form at physiological pHs.

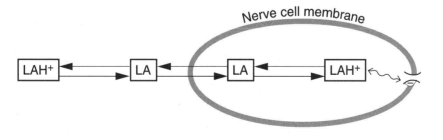

Figure 4-2. The unionized local anesthetic (LA) diffuses across the axon membrane and is converted to the ionized local anesthetic (LAH^+), which interacts with binding sites ($-$) in the sodium and potassium channels.

3. The **intermediate chain** determines how a local anesthetic is metabolized and can be either an ester or an amide.

    a. The **esters** are broken down by butyrylcholinesterases in the blood
        (1) **Cocaine** is only used for topical anesthesia.
        (2) **Procaine** (*Novocain*) is metabolized to para-aminobenzoic acid (PABA).
        (3) **Chloroprocaine** (*Nesacaine*) is metabolized most rapidly, has the shortest duration of action, and theoretically has the lowest risk of systemic toxicity.
        (4) **Tetracaine** (*Pontocaine*) is ten times as potent as procaine and ten times as toxic.

    b. The **amides,** which are metabolized by amidases in the liver, include:
        (1) **Lidocaine** (*Xylocaine*)
        (2) **Mepivacaine** (*Carbocaine*)
        (3) **Bupivacaine** (*Marcaine*)

C. **Toxic effects** are very uncommon but can be serious if the systemic absorption of the local anesthetic is excessive.

    1. **Myocardial depression** is due to sodium channel blockade in myocardial muscle.

    2. **Vasodilation** leads to a fall in blood pressure.

    3. **Anxiety or depression and convulsions** result from depressant actions on the CNS.

    4. **Hypersensitivity** reactions are rare and occur primarily with esters, which contain PABA derivatives.

D. **Epinephrine (EPI) is frequently combined with local anesthetics.**

    1. EPI reduces blood flow in the anesthetized area which:
        a. **Reduces bleeding,** making it useful during some types of surgeries.
        b. **Prolongs the anesthesia** by slowing the loss of anesthetic from the area of injection.
        c. **Reduces the systemic concentration** of the anesthetic, thereby lowering the incidence of toxicity.

    2. EPI is not used with cocaine, because cocaine by itself has vasoconstrictor activity, and it is not used on end-appendages where ischemia can be induced.

E. The symptoms of **local anesthetic toxicity must be treated** aggressively.

    1. **Oxygen** reduces the hypoxia.

    2. **Vasopressors or intravenous fluids** increase the blood pressure.

    3. **Diazepam** reduces the convulsions.

F. During spinal anesthesia, blood pressure may fall due to blockade of sympathetic pathways in the spinal cord.

V. SEDATIVE-HYPNOTIC AND ANTIANXIETY DRUGS

A. Hypnotics are medications that induce sleep and antianxiety drugs are medications that reduce anxiety and should have little hypnotic activity.

B. **The common mechanism of action is to enhance the inhibitory effects of gamma-aminobutyric acid (GABA) in the CNS.**

C. Side effects common to these drugs include:

    1. **Decreased REM sleep** with a rebound increase in REM sleep upon withdrawal

    2. **Drowsiness**

3. Hangover

4. **Tolerance** with prolonged administration due to:
   a. **Increased metabolism** from activation of mixed function oxidases (MFOs)
   b. **Reduced effects on the CNS**

5. **Respiratory depression.** These drugs reduce the sensitivity of the medullary respiratory centers to CO_2.
   a. The depression is increased when these drugs are combined with any other sedating drug.
   b. This is the **cause of death** from an overdose.
   c. **Tolerance does not develop to the depressant action on respiration.**
   d. The respiratory depression is very marked with the barbiturates and very weak with the benzodiazepines.

6. **Abuse potential. Physical dependence** occurs with all these drugs and results in an abstinence syndrome upon withdrawal.

D. **Benzodiazepine** preparations differ primarily in their duration of action.

   1. **Antianxiety preparations** usually have long durations of action ranging from twelve hours to several days. They include:
      a. **Chlordiazepoxide** (*Librium*)
      b. **Diazepam** (*Valium*)
      c. **Alprazolam** (*Xanax*)

   2. **Hypnotic preparations** (sleeping pills) have shorter durations of action than the antianxiety drugs.
      a. **Flurazepam** (*Dalmane*) has a short half-life, but active metabolites can lead to a long clinical effect, resulting in daytime drowsiness.
      b. **Temazepam** (*Restoril*) has a $t_{1/2}$ of 10 hours with no active metabolites.
      c. **Triazolam** (*Halcion*) has a short $t_{1/2}$ of 2.5 hours, which can result in early morning awakening.

   3. **All the benzodiazepines bind to benzodiazepine receptors,** which leads to an enhancement of GABA inhibition (Figure 4–3).

   4. **The effects** include:
      a. **Calming** of behavior
      b. **Reduction of anxiety**
      c. **Induction of sleep**
      d. **Anticonvulsant** actions
      e. **Muscle relaxation**

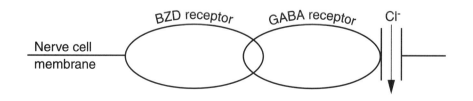

Figure 4-3. Relationship of the benzodiazepine (BZD) receptor to the gamma-aminobutyric acid (GABA) receptor. Enhanced chloride inflow will hyperpolarize (inhibit) CNS neurons, leading to sedative, antianxiety, and hypnotic effects.

5. There are no autonomic effects.

6. Side effects include:
  a. Drowsiness
  b. Dependence—long term use should be avoided
  c. Enhanced depression when combined with other CNS depressant drugs

7. The benzodiazepines have many **advantages over the barbiturates.**
  a. **Abuse is less common,** although it can occur.
  b. **Suicide potential is lower** due to the high therapeutic index (TI).
  c. **Less reduction of REM sleep** occurs.
  d. **The withdrawal syndrome is milder,** although much more prolonged.
  e. **Induction of MFOs is less pronounced.**
  f. **Flumazenil** (*Romazicon*), **a benzodiazepine antagonist,** will reverse the effects of the benzodiazepines.

E. Zolpidem (*Ambien*) is a hypnotic with little effect on the stages of sleep.

  1. Although it is **not a benzodiazepine,** it **binds to a subgroup of benzodiazepine receptors.**

  2. It is **antagonized by flumazenil.**

  3. It has little anxiolytic, anticonvulsant or muscle relaxant activity.

  4. The t½ is 2 hours.

F. **Chloral hydrate** (*Noctec*) **is a hypnotic prodrug** that is metabolized by alcohol dehydrogenase to the active moiety, trichloroethanol.

  1. **An unpleasant taste and odor** reduces the potential for abuse.

  2. **The TI is relatively low.**

G. Buspirone (*BuSpar*) is an antianxiety drug that:

  1. Is not a benzodiazepine

  2. Is a partial agonist at $5HT_{1A}$ receptors

  3. Does not have any abuse potential

  4. Has few CNS side effects (e.g., drowsiness is minimal)

H. Hydroxyzine (*Atarax,Vistaril*) is an antihistamine with:

  1. Antianxiety activity

  2. No abuse potential

  3. Marked sedative and anticholinergic effects

I. **Barbiturates** are derived from **barbituric acid,** a combination of urea and malonic acid.

  1. They are frequently provided as sodium salts (e.g., sodium pentobarbital) because the salt is more water soluble; however, it is very alkaline.

  2. **The barbiturates are classified by durations of action**
    a. **Ultrashort-acting barbiturates [e.g., thiopental** (*Pentothal*)**]** have very high lipid solubilities due to a sulphur in the structure. They are used as IV anesthetics.
    b. **Short- and intermediate-acting barbiturates [e.g. pentobarbital** (*Nembutal*)**]** have lower lipid solubilities and longer durations of action that are appropriate for sleeping pills.

   c. Long-acting barbiturates [e.g., phenobarbital (*Luminal*)] have the lowest lipid solubilities and the longest durations of action that are appropriate for sedatives or antianxiety drugs.

3. **Binding to plasma proteins** is highest for the highly lipid-soluble barbiturates.

4. **Metabolism by side chain oxidation** accounts for the clearance of all the barbiturates from the body. Only phenobarbital has some clearance (30%) by the kidney, and this can be increased by increasing the urinary pH.

5. **Acute intermittent porphyria is an absolute contraindication** for the use of the barbiturates.

6. **Patients who overdose on barbiturates develop respiratory depression** which is managed symptomatically by **assisting respiration** and stabilizing blood pressure.

J. **Clinical uses** of sedative–hypnotics and antianxiety drugs include:

1. **Treatment of anxiety or neuroses**

2. **Treatment of insomnia**

3. **Muscle relaxation**

4. **Treatment of seizures**

5 **Replacement therapy** during withdrawal from sedative–hypnotics (e.g., ethanol)

6. **IV anesthesia**

7. **Sedation before surgical procedures**

VI. CNS STIMULANTS

A. **Methylxanthines** [e.g., caffeine, theophylline (aminophylline), theobromine] have mild CNS stimulant effects.

1. The primary **mechanism of action** is controversial.
   a. **Adenosine receptors are blocked,** thereby decreasing the inhibitory actions of adenosine.
   b. **Phosphodiesterases are inhibited at high concentrations** which increases the concentration of intracellular cyclic AMP.

2. **Many effects** are induced, including:
   a. **CNS stimulation**
   b. **Myocardial stimulation**
   c. **Bronchodilation**
   d. **Diuresis**
   e. **Constriction of cerebral vessels,** which reduces headache

3. Caffeine is more effective on the CNS, and theophylline and theobromine are more effective at the peripheral sites.

B. **Amphetamines** are phenylethylamines.

1. **Absence of a catechol** in the structure allows for good penetration into the CNS.

2. The *d*-isomer of amphetamine is more potent on the CNS than the *l*-isomer.

3. Many **effects** occur, including:
   a. **Improvement of mood**
   b. **Increase in motor activity**
   c. **Reduction of appetite** which is temporary due to the rapid development of tolerance
   d. **Reduction of fatigue**

4. The actions are mediated, indirectly, through the release of endogenous catecholamines.

5. Appropriate indications include
   a. Hyperkinesis in children, especially with methylphenidate (*Ritalin*)
   b. Narcolepsy

6. An inappropriate indication is obesity.
   a. Amphetamine-like drugs have been used as diet products, however the reduction of appetite is temporary.
   b. Side effects, such as irritability, insomnia, and peripheral sympathetic activation can occur.

C. Convulsants act by many different mechanisms.

   1. Picrotoxin is a GABA receptor antagonist that blocks presynaptic inhibition (Site A in Figure 4–4).

   2. Strychnine is a glycine receptor antagonist that blocks postsynaptic inhibition (See Site B in Figure 4–4).

   3. Tetanus toxin blocks inhibitory, especially glycine, interneurons.

   4. Other convulsants increase excitatory transmission.

   5. Their only clinically important effect is respiratory stimulation, but they are not indicated for the treatment of respiratory depression from overdoses of sedative-hypnotics.

VII. ANTIPSYCHOTIC DRUGS

A. The typical antipsychotics block D_2 dopamine receptors in the limbic system which probably accounts for the therapeutic effects of these drugs in reducing the symptoms of psychoses (e.g., schizophrenia).

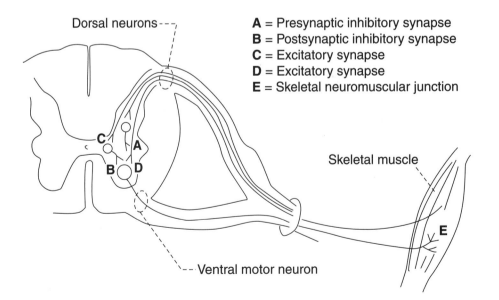

Figure 4-4. Neuronal pathways in the spinal cord.

B. Blockade at other sites leads to the sides effects.

   1. Blockade of D_2 receptors in the extrapyramidal system (basal ganglia) induces an iatrogenic parkinsonism.

      a. This complication can be reduced by anticholinergic drugs, such as benztropine (*Cogentin*).

      b. L-Dopa should not be used to treat antipsychotic-induced extrapyramidal symptoms.

   2. Blockade of D_2 receptors in the pituitary enhances the release of prolactin, which induces a galactorrhea.

   3. Blockade of histamine receptors leads to a sedation, but these drugs have no abuse potential and display no tolerance.

   4. Blockade of M-cholinoceptors leads to anticholinergic symptoms.

   5. Blockade of α-adrenoceptors induces hypotension.

   6. Serotonin (5-HT) receptors are also blocked.

   7. An action on the hypothalamus shifts body temperature towards the ambient temperature.

C. The drugs can be classified as:

   1. Typical drugs

      a. Phenothiazines include:

         (1) Chlorpromazine (*Thorazine*) and thioridazine (*Mellaril*) which are low potency phenothiazines.

         (2) Fluphenazine (*Prolixin*) which is a high potency phenothiazine.

      b. Thiothixene (*Navane*) and haloperidol are also high potency antipsychotics.

   2. Atypical drugs

      a. Risperidone (*Risperdal*) is a newer antipsychotic with $5HT_2$ receptor–blocking activity and fewer extrapyramidal symptoms than the typical antipsychotics.

      b. Clozapine (*Clozaril*) also blocks $5HT_2$ receptors. It:

         (1) Induces the fewest extrapyramidal symptoms

         (2) Is effective in some patients that are refractory to the typical antipsychotic drugs.

         (3) Can cause agranulocytosis.

      c. Olanzapine (*Zyprexa*) is similar to clozapine, but does not cause agranulocytosis.

D. The side effects are related to the potency.

   1. The high potency typical antipsychotics induce the most extrapyramidal symptoms.

   2. The low potency typical antipsychotics induce fewer extrapyramidal symptoms, but they induce more anticholinergic effects, more hypotension, and more sedation than the high potency typical antipsychotics.

   3. The TI is very large. At high doses, convulsions can rarely occur.

   4. Tardive dyskinesia is a major complication that can develop after long term administration of typical antipsychotics.

      a. Orofacial symptoms predominate.

      b. Withdrawal of the antipsychotic drug must be undertaken even though it can enhance the tardive dyskinesia.

   c. Anticholinergics do not reduce the tardive dyskinesia.

   d. One proposed theory is that tardive dyskinesia is due to an **up-regulation of the D_2 receptors** in the basal ganglia.

E. These drugs are **very long acting.**

   1. Binding to many tissues results in a **large V_d.**

   2. There are **many drug metabolites.**

F. **Antipsychotic drugs** are also used:

   1. as **antiemetics** due to an action to depress the chemoreceptor trigger zone.

   2. to treat many less common neurological disorders.

G. These drugs have been used as sedatives, although this is inappropriate in view of the risk of tardive dyskinesia.

VIII. LITHIUM CARBONATE

A. The only clinical indication for lithium is the treatment of **manic depressive illness (bipolar disorder),** including

   1. Acute treatment of the manic phase

   2. Acute treatment of the depressive phase

   3. Prophylaxis

B. A **delay of 7–10 days** occurs before lithium has a clinical effect.

C. **Side effects** are common if the blood lithium concentration gets into the toxic range, thus it is important to monitor the blood lithium concentrations to avoid toxicity.

   1. **Tremor** can develop and progress to convulsions.

   2. A **nephrogenic diabetes insipidus** can occur.

   3. There is **no specific antidote** for lithium.
      a. The thiazide diuretics will lead to lithium retention and enhance lithium toxicity; thus they should be avoided in patients being treated with lithium.
      b. A high sodium diet will increase lithium excretion.

D. Alternate drugs for bipolar depression are the anticonvulsants, carbamezepine (*Tegretol*) and valproic acid (*Depakene*)

IX. ANTIDEPRESSANTS

A. The primary clinical indication for antidepressants is **major depression (unipolar disorder).**

B. **Tricyclic antidepressants** have a structure that is similar to the phenothiazines.

   1. Imipramine, the prototype, also has many effects that are similar to the phenothiazines, however it
      a. Produces very **little D_2-receptor antagonism.**
      b. **Reduces amine reuptake,** which increases the concentration of NE and 5-HT in the CNS synapses.

   2. The onset of the antidepressant effect is delayed, taking **2–3 weeks** to develop; which supports a hypothesis that down-regulation of NE or 5-HT receptors may be necessary for the clinical effect to occur.

   3. These drugs **improve mood in depressed patients, but not in normal subjects,** which is the basis of the term "antidepressant".

4. **The side effects** vary among specific drugs (Table 4–2), but are generally similar to the phenothiazines. They include:
   a. Sedation
   b. **Anticholinergic effects,** such as tachycardia, arrhythmias, and blurred vision
   c. **Antiadrenergic effects,** such as orthostatic hypotension

5. Overdoses from tricyclics are common because depressed patients may ingest large amounts of the drug in an attempt to commit suicide. Treatment of an overdose involves:
   a. Supportive management
   b. Lidocaine to reduce arrhythmias
   c. Physostigmine to reverse anticholinergic effects

6. There are **other clinical uses** for the tricyclics.
   a. **Childhood enuresis** (bed-wetting) and **urinary incontinence** in the elderly can be reduced.
   b. Clomipramine (*Anafranil*) reduces obsessive-compulsive behaviors.

B. **Selective serotonin reuptake inhibitors (SSRIs)** inhibit serotonin reuptake but do not affect NE reuptake.

   1. Most new antidepressants, such as **fluoxetine** (*Prozac*), **sertraline** (*Zoloft*) and **paroxetine** (*Paxil*), are in this group.

   2. They are similar in efficacy to the tricyclics for the treatment of major depression.

   3. The main advantage is they are **much safer** due to a lack of:
      a. Sedation
      b. Hypotension
      c. Anticholinergic effects

   4. They can cause sexual dysfunction and CNS stimulation, leading to **insomnia.**

C. **Monoamine oxidase (MAO) inhibitors,** e.g., tranylcypromine (*Parnate*) and phenelzine (*Nardil*), are **competitive irreversible inhibitors of both MAO$_A$ and MAO$_B$.**

   1. This inhibition increases the concentrations of NE and other amines in the granules, which increases amine release.

   2. The MAO inhibitors **elevate mood in both normal and depressed people.**

   3. The side effects can be severe, including:
      a. Hepatotoxicity
      b. CNS stimulation
      c. Postural hypotension

Table 4-2
Magnitude of Side Effects from Tricyclic Antidepressants

	Sedation and anticholinergic activity
Doxepin (*Sinequan*)	High
Amitriptyline (*Elavil*)	High
Imipramine (*Tofranil*)	Moderate
Desipramine (*Norpramin*)	Low
Nortriptyline (*Aventyl, Pamelor*)	Low

d. Hypertensive crisis when taken with
   (1) **Foods containing tyramine,** such as cheeses, beans, pickled herring, beer, and wine
   (2) **Over-the-counter sympathomimetics**

4. Combinations of tricyclics and MAO inhibitors should be avoided because this can lead to excessive CNS stimulation.

X. DRUGS FOR PARKINSON'S DISEASE

A. **Parkinson's disease is due to a reduced dopamine (DA) content** in the cells of the **substantia nigra,** which leads to the symptoms of:

1. Tremor at rest

2. Cogwheel rigidity

3. Akinesia

4. Loss of postural reflexes

B. **Methylphenyltetrahydropyridine (MPTP) destroys DA neurons** and induces parkinsonian symptoms. It can be used to produce a valuable animal model.

C. **Treatments** for Parkinson's disease either increase DA effects or block ACh in the basal ganglia.

   1. **Levodopa** [L-dopa(*Dopar,Larodopa*)], the most effective treatment, is metabolized by dopa decarboxylase to DA, which increases the availability of DA, an inhibitory transmitter, in the basal ganglia.

   a. L-Dopa becomes effective in a few weeks, especially **for reducing the rigidity and akinesia.**

   b. L-Dopa is however **rapidly metabolized** in peripheral tissues, so that only 1% of the administered dose reaches the CNS.
      (1) **Pyridoxine (vitamin B$_6$) increases this metabolism** by activating dopa decarboxylase.
      (2) **Carbidopa** (*Sinemet*), **a peripheral dopa decarboxylase inhibitor** which slows the metabolism of L-dopa, is usually combined with L-dopa
         (a) The L-dopa dosage can then be reduced by 80% without changing the effectiveness.
         (b) The side effects from conversion of L-dopa to DA in the periphery are also reduced.

   c. Side effects from L-dopa include
      (1) **Nausea, vomiting, and anorexia** induced by stimulation of the chemoreceptor trigger zone. The severity of the nausea is reduced by gradually increasing the dose into the therapeutic range and by combining L-dopa with carbidopa.
      (2) **Postural hypotension**
      (3) **Arrhythmias** from actions of DA on the heart.
      (4) **Choreiform movements** due to excessive actions of DA on basal ganglion.
      (5) **Psychological disturbances** which can lead to insomnia and delirium.

   d. **ON-OFF effects** often develop after a year or more. These are indicative of "wearing off phenomena" at the end of dosage intervals and erratic effectiveness.

   e. **Contraindications** for L-dopa include:
      (1) **Treatment with MAO inhibitors,** because the combination can lead to a hypertensive crisis
      (2) **Glaucoma,** because L-dopa can induce a mydriasis

(3) Psychiatric disorders, especially those disorders being treated with antipsychotic drugs, which are DA antagonists.

2. DA receptor agonists have effects and side effects that are similar to L-dopa. They are often used with L-dopa and carbidopa to reduce the ON-OFF effects.

   a. **Bromocriptine** (*Parlodel*) and **pergolide** (*Permax*) are **non-selective DA agonists.**

   b. **Pramipexole** (*Mirapex*) and **ropinirole** (*Requip*) are **selective D_2 agonists,** which are very effective and have fewer side effects.

3. The **anticholinergics** [e.g., trihexyphenidyl (*Artane*), benztropine (*Cogentin*)] reduce the cholinergic excitatory tone in the basal ganglia.

   a. They are most frequently used in combination **with antipsychotic drugs** to reduce the extrapyramidal symptoms from the antipsychotic drugs.

   b. The side effects are due to central and peripheral cholinoceptor blockade.

4. Amantadine (*Symmetrel*) is an anti-viral drug that reduces the symptoms of Parkinson's disease. Tolerance to this therapeutic effect often develops within 6 months.

5. Antihistamines, such as diphenhydramine (*Benadryl*), do have some weak therapeutic effects which are probably due to the anticholinergic actions of these drugs.

6. Selegiline (*Eldepryl*) is a **MAO_B inhibitor.**

   a. **A slowing of the metabolism of DA** enhances the effectiveness of L-dopa.

   b. It can be used in combination with L-dopa, making it possible to lower the L-dopa dosage.

D. The order of efficacies of the available drugs for this disease is the following: L-dopa > bromocriptine > amantadine > anticholinergics

E. A common approach is to use the low efficacy drugs (e.g., selegiline, amantadine, anticholinergics) during the early stages of Parkinson's disease and reserve L-dopa with carbidopa and dopaminergic agonists for the later stages.

XI. DRUGS FOR HUNTINGTON'S DISEASE

A. **A loss of GABA or increased DA** in the basal ganglia leads to the choreiform movements that are characteristic of Huntington's disease. As a result, L-dopa and anticholinergics are inappropriate treatments.

B. **No treatment is very effective,** but some reduction of symptoms can be induced by DA depleters, antipsychotics (DA blockers) or cholinesterase inhibitors.

XII. ANTICONVULSANTS

A. **Animal models** are useful in the screening of potential drugs for the treatment of epilepsy.

   1. **The convulsant, pentylenetetrazol,** induces convulsions that have drug sensitivities similar to absence seizures.

   2. **Maximal electrical shock** induces convulsions with drug sensitivities similar to tonic-clonic seizures.

   3. **Kindling** from weak, long-term stimulation of the cortex or amygdala induces generalized seizures.

B. The anticonvulsants **act by reducing the excitability** of focal and **non-focal neurons** (primarily) by:

   1. **Enhancing GABA inhibition** which leads to an increased P_{Cl} and a hyperpolarization of neuronal membranes.

   2. **Prolonging sodium permeability inactivation** which enhances the effective refractory period of nerve cells

   3. **Blocking T-type calcium channels**

C. All sedative-hypnotic and antianxiety drugs have anticonvulsant activity, but most produce too much drowsiness (sedation) to be clinically useful.

D. **The selection** of a specific drug for treatment depends upon the **seizure type** (Table 4–3).

E. Each anticonvulsant has some unique features.

1. **Phenobarbital** (*Luminal*) has a half-life of 4 days. Patients develop some tolerance to the sedative-hypnotic effect, but not to the anti-epileptic effect.

2. **Primidone** (*Mysoline*) is an active drug and is also partially metabolized to phenobarbital, thus it has properties that are very similar to phenobarbital.

3. **Phenytoin** (*Dilantin*) is an effective anti-epileptic with no sedative activity.
   a. **Elimination follows zero-order kinetics.**
   b. **Gingival hyperplasia and cardiac arrhythmias** are important side effects.

4. **Carbamazepine** (*Tegretol*) is a tricyclic anticonvulsant which has **antidepressant** activity. A rare, but severe, side effect is **aplastic anemia.**

5. **Valproic acid** (*Depakene*) is useful for **many types of seizures.** It can be **hepatotoxic.**

6. **Ethosuximide** (*Zarontin*) is the drug of choice for **absence seizures.**

7. **Clonazepam** (*Klonopin*) is a benzodiazepine, which produces considerable sedation.

8. **Gabapentin** (*Neurontin*) is useful for partial seizures.

F. Many features are common to most antiepileptics.

1. None of these drugs are curative.

2. They tend to be **highly bound to plasma proteins.**

3. They are usually **cleared by hepatic metabolism.**
   a. They may **inhibit the metabolism** of other drugs.
   b. They may **induce the metabolism** of other drugs, e.g., the effectiveness of oral contraceptives can be reduced.
   c. It is important to measure the serum anticonvulsant concentration.

4. **Side effects** that usually occur, include:
   a. **CNS depression** (Even phenytoin induces a lethargy.)
   b. **Skin rashes**
   c. **Nystagmus**
   d. **Teratogenicity**

Table 4-3
Activities of Anticonvulsants for Specific Seizure Patterns

	Tonic-clonic	Partial	Absence	Akinetic and atonic
Phenobarbital (*Luminal*)	+	+		
Primidone (*Mysoline*)	+	+		
Phenytoin (*Dilantin*)	++	++	$\ominus$	
Carbamazepine (*Tegretol*)	++	++		
Valproic acid (*Depakene*)	+	+	++	+
Ethosuximide (*Zarontin*)			++	
Clonazepam (*Klonopin*)			+	+

Note: (–) means exacerbated

G. **Status epilepticus** is a life-threatening disorder for which therapy must be initiated rapidly.

  1. **An intravenous benzodiazepine,** such as diazepam (*Valium*) or lorazepam (*Ativan*), is the treatment of choice.

  2. If the benzodiazepine is ineffective, other measures must be tried, including:
  - **a.** **Phenytoin, given intravenously**
  - **b.** **Phenobarbital, given intravenously**
  - **c.** General anesthesia

XIII. ANALGESIC ANTIPYRETICS

A. All the analgesic antipyretics act by **inhibiting cyclooxygenase** (COX) thereby reducing prostaglandin synthesis.

B. **Aspirin** (acetylsalicylic acid) is a salicylate that acetylates and **irreversibly inhibits COX-1 and COX-2.** New COX must be synthesized to recover from the effects of aspirin.

  1. The major **therapeutic effects** include:
  - **a.** **Mild analgesia,** due to reduced prostaglandin synthesis at the sensory nerve endings.
  - **b.** **Antipyresis,** due to reduced prostaglandin synthesis in the hypothalamic temperature control center. This reduces an elevated body temperature.
  - **c.** **Anti-inflammatory** actions at high doses, due to reduced prostaglandins at the sites of inflammation.

  2. These effects occur without tolerance and without euphoria.

  3. **Side effects** from aspirin include:
  - **a.** **Gastric ulcerations** and gastric hemorrhaging, which can be **increased by ingesting ethanol**
  - **b.** **Inhibition of platelet aggregation.** This adverse effect is taken advantage of during the management of patients:
    - **(1)** After a myocardial infarction
    - **(2)** With transient ischemic attacks
    - **(3)** With angina, especially unstable angina
    - **(4)** With atrial fibrillation
  - **c.** **Hypersensitivity** reactions that:
    - **(1)** Are not immunologically mediated
    - **(2)** May be due to increased **leukotrienes**
  - **d.** **Reduced renal uric acid secretion at low doses** and reduced uric acid reabsorption (uricosuria) at high doses
  - **e.** **Reye's syndrome** in children with chicken pox (varicella) or influenza viral infections. Aspirin is best avoided in children.

  4. Aspirin induces **acute toxic effects** in the following order as the dose is increased from the therapeutic to the toxic range.
  - **a.** **Tinnitus** is an early indicator of toxicity.
  - **b.** **Uncoupling of oxidative phosphorylation** increases CO_2 production, which increases respiration.
  - **c.** **Direct medullary stimulation** also enhances respiration, leading to respiratory alkalosis and HCO_3 excretion (loss).
  - **d.** **Acidosis** subsequently occurs as a result of:
    - **(1)** **Direct respiratory depression**
    - **(2)** **Acidic products** of aspirin metabolism. This leads to a fluid and electrolyte loss.
    - **(3)** **Previous loss of** HCO_3

    5. **Management** of aspirin overdoses involves:
      a. **Emesis or lavage**
      b. **Fluids with HCO$_3$**
      c. **Monitoring the blood aspirin concentration** beginning 6 hours after ingestion

C. **Acetaminophen** (*Tylenol*) also inhibits COX, especially in the CNS.

    1. The primary **effects** of acetaminophen however, are quite different from aspirin, and include:
      a. **Mild analgesic activity**
      b. **Antipyretic activity**
      c. **No anti-inflammatory activity**
      d. **None of the side effects of aspirin**

    2. **The major adverse effect** from high doses is a **delayed hepatic necrosis.**
      a. A toxic phase 1 metabolite builds up in the liver because of the **depletion of glutathione.**
      b. This toxicity is especially prominent in combination with ethanol.
      c. The hepatotoxicity can be avoided by early administration of **N-acetylcysteine,** which replenishes the stores of glutathione.

D. **Ibuprofen** (*Motrin, Nuprin, Advil*) and **naproxen (*Aleve*) reversibly inhibit COX** and have:

    1. Effects that are very **similar to aspirin,** including
      a. **Mild analgesic activity.** Ibuprofen is especially effective for dysmenorrhea.
      b. **Antipyretic activity**
      c. **Anti-inflammatory activity**

    2. **Side effects** that are similar to, but milder than, the side effects for aspirin, including:
      a **Gastrointestinal bleeding**
      b. **Increased bleeding times**
      c. **Overdose toxicity like aspirin**

E. **Ketorolac** (*Toradol*) is an unusual NSAID, in that it can be **given intramuscularly** as well as orally.

    1. It is only used for the **treatment of acute pain.**

    2. It has a clinical efficacy similar to morphine.

XIV. NARCOTIC ANALGESICS

A. **The prototype, morphine,** is extracted from the opium poppy in which 10% of the alkaloid content is morphine and 1% is codeine.

B. Morphine and codeine can be modified to form semisynthetic derivatives, including:

    1. Heroin (diacetylmorphine), which is more lipid soluble and has a more rapid onset of action

    2. Oxycodone (*Roxicodone*)

C. Many synthetic narcotics have also been produced, such as:

    1. Meperidine (*Demerol*)

    2. Levorphanol (*Levo-Dromoran*)

    3. Methadone (*Dolophine*)

    4. Fentanyl (*Sublimaze*)

    5. Propoxyphene (*Darvon, Dolene*)

D. The properties of morphine are representative of most of the drugs in this class.

    1. Morphine is **quite lipid soluble**.

        a. Absorption from the gut is good, but the serum morphine concentration is **variable** due to first-pass metabolism by the liver.

        b. The drug distributes in the total body water.

        c. It is **metabolized by glucuronide conjugation.**

        d. Parenteral administration is commonly used to induce a rapid, predictable analgesic effect.

    2. The binding sites for morphine are the endorphin, dynorphin, and enkephalin receptors. **Mu, kappa and delta receptor subtypes** have been identified.

    3. Morphine induces many pharmacological **effects.**

        a. Analgesia occurs due to a decrease of pain perception and a decrease in the psychological response to pain.

            (1) An **inhibitory** action **on substance P release** in the spinal cord (Figure 4–5), may account for some of the analgesic effects.

            (2) This is accompanied by a **mental clouding** or drowsiness.

            (3) Although the first dose can be dysphoric, subsequent doses produce a euphoria.

        b. Respiratory depression is induced by a reduction in the sensitivity of the medullary respiratory centers to CO_2. This occurs with all the narcotic analgesics and is the primary **cause of death** from an acute overdose.

        c. Physical dependence and tolerance occur with long term use, which means that a withdrawal syndrome will develop when the drug is discontinued. Cross-tolerance occurs with all other narcotic analgesics.

        d. Antitussive (cough suppressant) actions are prominent.

        e. An emetic action is often observed with the initial doses.

        f. Miosis is induced by increased parasympathetic tone to the pupil. This is less pronounced with meperidine due to an anticholinergic effect.

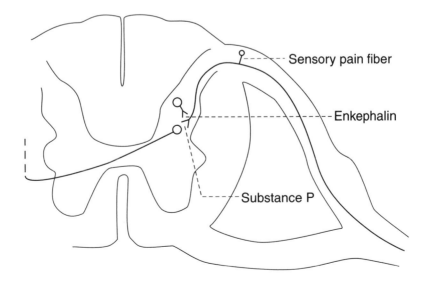

Figure 4-5.   Presynaptic inhibition by enkephalins on substance P release in the spinal pain pathway.

     g. **Constipation** results from decreased GI motility, even though there is an increased tone of the GI smooth muscle.

     h. **Histamine release** can be induced.

     i. **Tone of the biliary tract and ureters** can be increased.

E. **Narcotic antagonists** have a structure that is very similar to morphine (Figure 4–6). A bulky substitution on the nitrogen results in antagonistic actions.

    1. The **pure antagonists** have no analgesic activity.

      a. **Naloxone** (*Narcan*) will:

        (1) **Reverse the respiratory depression** from an overdose of a narcotic

        (2) Not affect the respiratory depression from a sedative-hypnotic

        (3) **Induce a withdrawal syndrome** in a narcotic addict

      b. **Naltrexone** (*Revia*) **is more effective orally** and has a **longer duration of action** than naloxone.

    2. The **weak agonist/antagonist analgesics,** such as **pentazocine** (*Talwin*), have analgesic activity in addition to antagonistic activity.

      a. They **will not reverse the respiratory depression** caused by a narcotic.

      b. They will **induce a withdrawal syndrome** in a narcotic addict.

      c. Most new narcotic analgesics are in this group. The rationale behind their use is that these analgesics should be abused less and should have less respiratory depression.

F. **Therapeutic uses** of the narcotic analgesics include:

    1. **Analgesia**

      a. Morphine is more potent than codeine, which is more potent than aspirin.

      b. Narcotics are used primarily for short term analgesia (e.g., myocardial infarction), except in terminal patients. The analgesic antipyretics are preferred to reduce chronic pain.

    2. **Diarrhea.** **Diphenoxylate** with atropine (*Lomotil*) or **loperamide** (*Imodium*) are preferred as they have few CNS effects.

    3. **Neuroleptic anesthesia** (e.g., fentanyl)

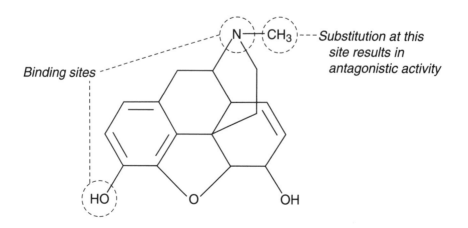

Figure 4-6. Modification of the narcotic structure (at N) results in the narcotic antagonists. This diagram shows the structure of morphine.

4. **Antitussive** activity

   a. **Codeine** induces more cough suppression than morphine.

   b. **Dextromethorphan** (*Benylin DM*) has little narcotic activity, but it does have cough suppressant activity.

5. **Reduction of narcotic withdrawal symptoms.** This requires a drug, such as **methadone,** with a long duration of action.

6. **Maintenance of a narcotic addict,** using methadone

G. **Clinical uses of the narcotic antagonists** include:

1. **Analgesia** with the agonist/antagonist analgesics

2. **Treatment of the respiratory depression from an acute narcotic overdose** using naloxone

3. **Diagnosis of physical dependence** to a narcotic. Naloxone will precipitate an abstinence syndrome in narcotic addicts.

4. **Management of a narcotic addict.** Naltrexone will reduce the euphoric effects of the narcotics.

5. **Management of an alcoholic.** Naltrexone reduces the craving for ethanol.

5

Substance Abuse

I. GENERAL FEATURES

A. Drugs are abused primarily to induce a **feeling of euphoria.**

B. Abuse of a drug is often, but not always, associated with kinetic, dynamic, homeostatic or learned **tolerance.**

C. **An acute tolerance** (with first dose) has been described for ethanol.

D. **Cross-tolerance** occurs between drugs with the same mechanism of action.

E. Repeated drug use may also lead to **psychological dependence, physical dependence and cross-dependence** (between drugs with the same mechanism of action). A dopaminergic pathway in the CNS may be involved in the desire to use drugs of abuse.

F. The symptoms during withdrawal tend to mirror (be the opposite of) those from drug administration.

G. Withdrawal from a drug of abuse is usually less severe with long-acting drugs than with short-acting drugs within the same class. This is the theoretical basis for replacement therapy.

H. Abusers of drugs usually derive more pleasure from a drug with a rapid onset of action than from a drug with a slow onset of action within the same class.

II. SEDATIVE-HYPNOTICS

A. **Ethanol** is a commonly abused legal substance.

   1. Due to **high lipid solubility and high water solubility,** ethanol distributes in the total body water.

   2. Clearance from the body occurs in the liver.

      a. **Metabolism** by the **alcohol and aldehyde dehydrogenases** (Figure 5–1) follows zero-order kinetics.

         (1) The products are acetaldehyde and acetic acid.

         (2) Two molecules of NADH are produced for each molecule of ethanol.

      b. An insignificant amount is metabolized by mixed function oxidases (MFOs), but this can induce the MFOs.

   3. The effects of ethanol are related to the blood ethanol concentration.

      a. **The legal limit** for driving in most states is **80 mg% (80 mg/100 ml).**

      b. **Death** due to respiratory depression occurs in the range of **500 mg%,** although this is quite variable.

      c. **Treatment** of an overdose of ethanol is **symptomatic.**

   4. **Acute adverse effects** develop after a single exposure to ethanol.

      a. **Behavior is changed** due to a loss of inhibitions.

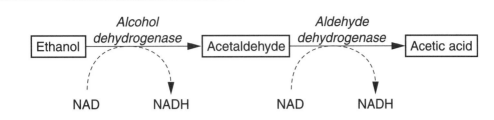

Figure 5-1. Metabolism of ethanol. *NAD*=nicotinamide adenine dinucleotide; *NADH*=reduced nicotinamide adenine dinucleotide

    b. The effects of other CNS depressants are enhanced.
    c. **Hypothermia** results from a peripheral vasodilation, which makes a person feel warm even though body heat is being lost.
    d. **Hangovers** are common after drinking ethanol, and may represent symptoms of an acute withdrawal.

5. **Adverse effects from chronic (repeated) use** occur on almost every tissue in the body and include:
    a. **Physical and psychological dependence**
    b. **Activation of MFOs,** which increases the metabolism of many other drugs (e.g., phenytoin, warfarin)
    c. **Edema**
    d. **Hypertension**
    e. **Cardiomyopathy**
    f. **Liver damage** (e.g., cirrhosis)
    g. **Changes in blood glucose**
    h. **Damage to the gastrointestinal tract**
    i. **Anemias**
    j. **Malnutrition, especially thiamine deficiency** which leads to the Wernicke-Korsakoff syndrome
    k. **Psychological depression**
    l. **Fetal alcohol syndrome.** Ethanol is a common cause of birth defects

6. A low intake of ethanol (one drink per day) increases HDL and decreases LDL cholesterol. This may reduce the risk of heart disease.

7. **Withdrawal** from ethanol in someone who is dependent leads to a **stimulatory syndrome** which lasts about one week.
    a. **Tremor, hallucinations, convulsions and delirium tremens** can occur during withdrawal.
    b. It is important to **replace thiamine** and improve the diet.
    c. The severity of the withdrawal symptoms can be reduced by **replacement therapy with an antianxiety drug** (e.g., diazepam or chlordiazepoxide).

8. Long-term treatment of a recovering alcoholic requires counseling and group support therapy. Naltrexone can reduce the craving for ethanol.

9. **Disulfiram** (*Antabuse*) is occasionally useful to help alcoholics avoid the use of ethanol.
    a. It **inhibits the enzyme, aldehyde dehydrogenase.**
    b. **An accumulation of acetaldehyde** leads to a toxic syndrome whenever ethanol is ingested.

10. Methanol has intoxicating effects similar to ethanol, except it is much more toxic.

    a. Metabolism by alcohol and aldehyde dehydrogenases results in the production of **formaldehyde and formic acid.**

        (1) **Acidosis** is the cause of death from acute ingestion.

        (2) **Retinal nerve damage** leads to blindness.

    b. **The specific antidote** for the treatment of methanol intoxication is **ethanol,** which competes with methanol at the metabolic enzymes and slows the production of the toxic metabolites.

11. Ethylene glycol is metabolized by the same pathway to products which cause acidosis and renal failure. An acute intoxication is treated in a manner similar to methanol intoxication.

B. Barbiturates, e.g., **pentobarbital and secobarbital,** are very common drugs of abuse, although any sedative-hypnotic or antianxiety drug can be abused.

    1. These drugs produce a **CNS depression with euphoria,** reduction of anxiety, and drowsiness, which is similar to the effects of ethanol.

        a. **Tolerance** occurs, but it is not large (5–10 times)

        b. **Cross-tolerance** develops to alcohol, barbiturates, general anesthetics, benzodiazepines, and other sedative-hypnotics.

    2. An overdose leads to **respiratory depression,** which should be treated symptomatically.

    3. **Barbiturate withdrawal can be severe** and life-threatening with:

        a. A prolonged delirium

        b. Grand mal convulsions

    4. **Substitution therapy** (e.g., phenobarbital, given orally) can be used to reduce the withdrawal symptoms. The phenobarbital is then slowly withdrawn.

C. Benzodiazepines have effects that are similar to other sedative-hypnotics.

    1. They are less subject to abuse than the barbiturates.

    2. When they are abused, the withdrawal syndrome is very mild, but very long in duration.

D. Inhalants are most commonly used by very young abusers.

    1. Inhalation of vapors from solvents, glue, gasoline, or anesthetics induces effects that are also very similar to ethanol.

    2. As with other halogenated hydrocarbons, hepatotoxicity, cardiac toxicity, and carcinogenicity can occur.

III. OPIOIDS

A. Heroin, used intravenously, is the most popular opioid for abuse.

B. The initial dose may be unpleasant with nausea, but subsequent doses induce a rush, euphoria, a reduction of anxiety, and contentment in the abuser.

C. **Marked tolerance** (up to 1000 times) to the desired effects occurs with repeated use of the opioids.

D. **Common causes of death** in heroin addicts are:

    1. **Respiratory depression** from an overdose. This can be reversed with naloxone.

    2. Infections from using unsterilized needles and syringes

E. The withdrawal syndrome, which begins in 6 hours and peaks in 48 hours, includes:

    1. Nausea, vomiting, diarrhea and sweating.

    2. Restlessness and tremor

F. Withdrawal from heroin can be performed by:

    1. "Cold turkey" (provide only symptomatic treatment)

    2. Replacement therapy with methadone

    3. Treatment with clonidine to reduce the symptoms

G. After withdrawal, abusers need long-term **rehabilitation** with

    1. Group therapy

    2. Methadone maintenance, which induces tolerance so no effect is obtained from heroin

    3. Depot naltrexone

IV. CIGARETTES

A. Nicotine is the active substance and is responsible for the addictive nature of cigarettes.

    1. Stimulation of the CNS induces arousal, relaxation, and a mild euphoria.

    2. Activation of the sympathetic nervous system induces a vasoconstriction and an increase in blood pressure.

B. The tars and carbon monoxide inhaled increase the risk of:

    1. Chronic obstructive pulmonary disease (COPD)

    2. Cancer

    3. Heart disease

C. Physical and psychological dependence occurs. Abstinence leads to anxiety, insomnia, and enhanced appetite which can last for several months.

D. Many approaches are available which slightly increase the probability of successfully abstaining from cigarettes.

    1. Nicotine is available in a patch, in gum, and in an inhaler.

    2. Bupropion (*Zyban*) is an antidepressant that has been introduced as an aid to stop smoking.

    3. Behavioral modification programs are also helpful.

V. CNS STIMULANTS

A. Cocaine and amphetamines are the most commonly abused CNS stimulants.

B. The magnitude of the euphoria depends on the speed of onset.

    1. Amphetamines are usually taken orally, which results in a **slow onset.**

    2. Cocaine can be ingested, chewed, snorted, injected, or smoked (as crack in the free base form). **Crack** that is smoked has the most **rapid onset** and induces the most pleasurable effects.

C. They produce a **euphoria** with:

1. Enhanced self-confidence and alertness

2. Increased motor activity

3. **Little physical dependence.** Fatigue is the primary physical symptom during withdrawal.

4. **Strong psychological dependence.**

D. The period of euphoria varies depending on the half-life of the drug in the body.

1. **Cocaine induces** a **very short euphoria** (approximately 15 minutes) that is followed by a period of **marked dysphoria.**

2. The euphoria from amphetamines has a much longer duration.

E. Chronic abusers develop **paranoid, psychotic-like** symptoms.

F. Overdoses can be dangerous.

1. **Sympathomimetic actions** can lead to **tachycardia and arrhythmias.**

2. Abusers can become **aggressive** and experience **hallucinations.**

3. **Cocaine** can also induce:
   a. **Gangrene,** due to a peripheral vasoconstriction
   b. **Perforation of the nasal septum,** due to vasoconstriction in the nasal mucosa
   c. **Convulsions,** due to local anesthetic effects on the brain

VI. HALLUCINOGENS

A. These are drugs that **induce visual hallucinations.**

1. **Lysergic acid diethylamide (LSD),** psilocin, and harmaline are **indole** hallucinogens.
   a. The indole structure in these substances also occurs in serotonin.
   b. They may act by blocking serotonin receptors.

2. **Mescaline** and MDMA (methylenedioxymethamphetamine, **ecstasy**) are **phenylethylamine** hallucinogens.
   a. The phenylethylamines have more **sympathomimetic** effects than the indoles.
   b. MDMA is often used to decrease fatigue and enhance awareness at rave parties.

3. **No physical dependence** occurs.

4. **Cross-tolerance** occurs between the indole and phenylethylamine hallucinogens.

5. Overdoses can result in a state of panic and psychotic behavior. These symptoms can be treated with diazepam.

B. Phencyclidine (PCP)

1. PCP, or "angel dust," is structurally similar to the anesthetic ketamine.

2. Although it produces hallucinations, there is **no cross-tolerance with LSD.**

3. Low doses induce a **drunken-like state.**

4. High doses produce an **amphetamine-like state** in which the abuser can become very physically aggressive and difficult to control; thus it is a very dangerous drug.

VII. MARIJUANA

A. The hemp plant is the source of marijuana, which contains the active ingredient, **Δ^9tetrahydrocannabinol (Δ^9THC).** It is usually abused by smoking.

1. Δ^9THC is **very lipid soluble** and traces remain in the body for days after use.

2. Metabolism to an active product, 11-OH-Δ^9THC, occurs in the liver. This product is further hydroxylated to an inactive metabolite, 8,11-OH$_2$-Δ^9THC.

B. A vivid dream-like state is induced with some **motor incoordination** and a **loss of sense of time.** Hallucinations can occur at high doses.

C. Chronic use leads to **some tolerance** for these effects, **apathy, and chronic bronchitis.**

D. Dronabinol (*Marinol*), which is Δ^9THC, has **antiemetic** activity that is useful during cancer chemotherapy.

VIII. ANABOLIC STEROIDS

A. Steroids are often inappropriately used to enhance athletic performance.

B. The Anabolic Steroid Control Act of 1990 made such use illegal.

6

Autacoids, Drugs for Inflammatory Disorders, and Vitamins

I. HISTAMINE

A. Histamine is an autacoid that is present in mast cells and circulating basophils. Autacoids are substances that function as local hormones or neuromodulators in the body.

B. Histamine **acts on H_1 and H_2 receptors** at many sites in the body.

    1. The important pharmacological effects of histamine are listed in Table 6–1.

    2. A **triple response** is induced after intradermal injection.
        a. A **direct vasodilation** produces a localized **red spot** at the site of injection.
        b. **Activation of nerve endings** induces an axon reflex that produces a vasodilation and a **flare.**
        c. **Increased capillary permeability** induces a **wheal** at the site of the red spot.

C. The **clinical uses** of histamine are of minor importance.

    1. **Achlorhydria** after the administration of histamine is useful for diagnosing **pernicious anemia.** The treatment for pernicious anemia is **vitamin B_{12} (cyano-cobalamin).**

    2. Supersensitivity to histamine can be useful for the **diagnosis of asthma.**

II. HISTAMINE BLOCKERS

A. Allergic disorders can be treated with histamine blockers.

B. The effects of endogenous histamine release can be blocked by several classes of drugs.

    1. **Cromolyn** (*Intal*) **reduces mast cell degranulation.**
        a. The release of all mast cell mediators, including histamine, is decreased.
        b. **Inhalation** of the dry powder or aerosol is the usual route of administration, because cromolyn is not absorbed after oral administration.
        c. The primary clinical use of cromolyn is the **prophylactic treatment of asthma and allergic disorders.**

    2. **H_1 antihistamines are competitive antagonists** at H_1 receptors. Drugs in this class include diphenhydramine (*Benadryl*), dimenhydrinate (*Dramamine*), chlorpheniramine (*Chlor-Trimeton, Teldrin*), and meclizine (*Antivert*).
        a. On-going histamine effects are only weakly reduced, thus the H_1-antihistamines work best if administered before exposure to an allergen.

Table 6–1
Effects of Histamine

Receptors	Effects
H_1 & H_2	Vasodilates arterioles and venules (leads to hypotension and shock)
H_1 & H_2	Increases capillary permeability (leads to edema)
H_1	Contracts bronchial and intestinal smooth muscle
H_1	Acts on sensory nerve endings to cause pain and itching
H_2	Increases heart rate and contractility
H_2	Increases gastric secretions

    b. The activity versus acute allergic reactions is better than the activity versus chronic allergies.

    c. There are many **clinical uses** for H_1 antihistamines, including treatment of:

        (1) Seasonal allergic rhinitis

        (2) Acute urticaria

        (3) Anxiety

        (4) Insomnia

        (5) Nausea

        (6) Parkinson's disease

    d. The **side effects** include:

        (1) Sedation

        (2) **Anticholinergic symptoms,** such as constipation, urinary retention, and dry mouth

    e. The second-generation H_1-antihistamines [e.g., loratadine (*Claritin*)] do not have these side effects.

    3. The **H_2 antihistamines** [e.g., cimetidine (*Tagamet*)] act primarily to reduce gastric secretions and are used to treat **peptic ulcer disease** (See Chapter 2 XII A 2). They have no effects on H_1 receptors.

III. EICOSANOIDS

    A. This large group of autacoids is **widely distributed** in the body.

    B. They are locally synthesized (Figure 6–1) and released as needed **(de novo synthesis).**

    C. The synthesis of prostacyclin (PGI_2), prostaglandins and thromboxane (TXA_2) is reduced by aspirin and the NSAIDs, which inhibit the enzyme cyclooxygenase. The NSAIDs have no effect on lipoxygenase.

    D. The eicosanoids have very **short durations** of action (approximately 1 minute) and induce **many effects.**

        1. Prostaglandin E_2 (PGE_2) or dinoprostone (*Prostin E2*) and $PGF_{2\alpha}$ or carboprost (*Prostin 15M*) **increase uterine activity.**

        a. They can be used to **induce labor and abortions.**

        b. Ibuprofen, by blocking prostaglandin synthesis, reduces the symptoms of dysmenorrhea.

        2. Prostaglandin E_1 (PGE_1) or alprostadil (*Prostin VR*) can be used to relax vascular smooth muscle and **maintain a patent ductus arteriosus.** Indomethacin, by blocking prostaglandin synthesis, induces closure of the ductus arteriosus.

        3. PGE **bronchodilates** and PGF **bronchoconstricts.**

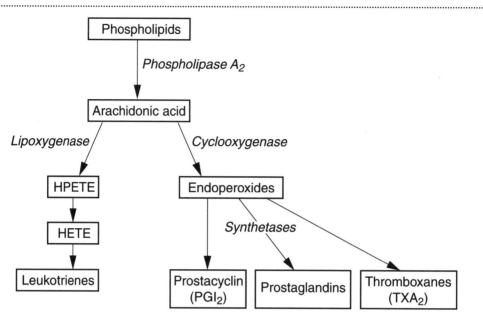

Figure 6–1. Synthesis of the eicosanoids. *HPETE*=hydroperoxyeicosatetraenoic acid; *HETE*=hydroxyeicosatetraenoic acid

4. PGE and PGI$_2$ **decrease gastric acid secretions. Misoprostol** (*Cytotec*) is a PGE$_1$ derivative that is used to **reduce gastric ulcerations from the NSAIDs.**

5. PGE and PGI$_2$ **sensitize afferent nerve endings to pain.**

6. Eicosanoids also have circulatory effects.
  a. TXA$_2$ from platelets and PGI$_2$ from vessel walls are important local hormones in the **control of the microcirculation** (Figure 6–2).
  b. PGI$_2$ or epoprostenol (*Flolan*) vasodilates and can be administered from an IV infusion pump to **treat primary pulmonary hypertension.**
  c. Alprostadil injected into the penis causes a vasodilation and induces a **penile erection. Sildenafil** (*Viagra*), not an eicosanoid, is an oral drug that **enhances penile erections by inhibiting phosphodiesterase type 5** and thereby dilating blood vessels in the penis.

IV. DRUGS FOR MIGRAINE HEADACHES

A. An initial intracranial vasoconstriction is followed by a prolonged extracranial vasodilation during which the migraine headache occurs.

B. **Acute treatment** involves:

  1. **Mild analgesics** for weak migraines.

  2. **Ergotamine,** often combined with caffeine (*Cafergot*), to induce a **direct vasoconstriction.** It is only used acutely because of the toxicity associated with chronic administration (e.g., prolonged vasoconstriction can result in gangrene).

  3. **Sumatriptan** (*Imitrex*) which **vasoconstricts by activating 5-HT$_1$ receptors.** Although safer than ergotamine, there is a risk of inducing a coronary vasospasm in patients with coronary artery disease.

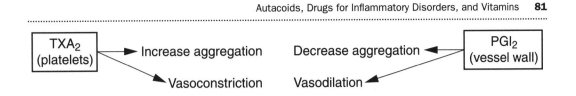

Figure 6–2. Local hormonal control of the microcirculation by thromboxane (TXA$_2$) in the platelets and prostacyclin (PGI$_2$) in the vessel wall.

    C. Prophylaxis can be obtained with:

       1. β-blockers or calcium channel blockers

       2. Methysergide (*Sansert*), **a partial 5-HT agonist,** which has a delayed onset

V. ANTIASTHMATIC DRUGS

    A. Asthma appears to be caused by an **inflammation of the airways** with **bronchoconstriction, bronchial wall edema, and increased respiratory secretions.**

    B. Methacholine and histamine induce a bronchoconstriction and can be used as **provocative** diagnostic tests for asthma, although these tests can be dangerous.

    C. The sympathomimetics relieve the acute symptoms of asthma by **β$_2$-mediated bronchodilation** and by reducing mediator release from the mast cells.

       1. Ephedrine is a weak sympathomimetic. Tolerance to the clinical effect can also develop.

       2. Epinephrine (*Adrenalin*) induces β$_2$ effects.

          a. It also has α-agonistic effects that **reduce airway congestion.**

          b. Cardiovascular side effects, such as **increased blood pressure, heart rate, and myocardial contractility,** can be very pronounced.

          c. Epinephrine is the **treatment of choice for acute anaphylaxis.**

       3. Isoproterenol (*Isuprel*) has much weaker actions on α-receptors than epinephrine and induces more vasodilation.

          a. Increases in heart rate and contractility can be very large, due to:

             (1) β$_1$ Effects on the heart

             (2) Reflexly mediated increases in sympathetic tone induced by the fall in blood pressure from the β$_2$-vasodilation.

          b. Repeated administration can result in an **anomalous bronchoconstriction.**

          c. The duration of action is **short** due to a rapid metabolism.

       4. Terbutaline (*Bricanyl, Brethine*), **albuterol** (*Proventil, Ventolin*) and **metaproterenol** (*Alupent*) are relatively **selective β$_2$ agonists** with only weak effects on β$_1$ and α-receptors.

          a. A **reflex-induced tachycardia** will occur, due to a fall in blood pressure.

          b. A **skeletal muscle tremor** is the most common side effect.

          c. The non-catecholamine structure leads to a much **slower metabolism, a longer duration of action, and greater oral efficacy.**

       5. Salmeterol (*Serevent*) is a **long-acting β$_2$ agonist** that can be used for prophylaxis.

    D. The **glucocorticoids** are potent anti-inflammatory drugs that have the highest efficacy in the treatment of asthma.

       1. They **reduce the inflammation** in the airways and enhance the β$_2$ effects of sympathetic activation on the airways.

2. Long term administration of the systemic glucocorticoids leads to **many side effects, including adrenal suppression, ulcers, and osteoporosis.**

3. Beclomethasone (*Beclovent, Vanceril*) is a very effective **inhaled** glucocorticoid.
  a. Any drug that reaches the circulation is rapidly metabolized.
  b. The blood concentrations remain low and there are **fewer side effects** than with the systemic glucocorticoids.

E. Cromolyn (*Intal*) stabilizes mast cells, probably by reducing the calcium influx during mast cell degranulation.

  1. **Mediator release is reduced.**

  2. The onset of action is very slow, so it can only be used **for prophylaxis.**

F. Theophylline (*Slo-Bid, Theo-Dur*) **blocks adenosine receptors.** It also inhibits phosphodiesterases, which increases the concentration of cyclic adenosine monophosphate (cAMP); however, this does not occur at therapeutic concentrations.

  1. The rate of metabolism of theophylline in the liver is quite variable between patients (e.g., smokers metabolize it faster than non-smokers).

  2. **The side effects** can be pronounced.
    a. **CNS stimulation** can progress to convulsions.
    b. **Tachycardia and arrhythmias** can occur.
    c. Rapid IV injections are dangerous due to marked cardiovascular effects.

  3. The blood theophylline concentrations should be monitored, because theophylline has a low therapeutic index.

G. Ipratropium (*Atrovent*) is an **inhaled quaternary anticholinergic.**

  1. **Muscarinic blockade** results in bronchodilation and reduced respiratory secretions.

  2. There are **no systemic anticholinergic effects** because it is not absorbed after inhalation.

H. Zafirlukast (*Accolate*), a **leukotriene antagonist,** and **zileuton** (*Zyflo*), a **lipoxygenase inhibitor,** are also effective for the treatment of asthma.

VI. DRUGS FOR RHEUMATOID ARTHRITIS

A. Rheumatoid arthritis is an inflammatory disorder involving many organs in the body, including the joints.

B. Aspirin at high dosages has anti-inflammatory activity that reduces the symptoms of rheumatoid arthritis.

  1. The high dosages also saturate the metabolic enzymes and prolong the duration of action of aspirin.

  2. The most common side effects are **gastric irritation and GI bleeding.**

C. Other nonsteroidal anti-inflammatory drugs (NSAIDs), such as indomethacin (*Indocin*), tolmetin (*Tolectin*), ibuprofen (*Motrin*), sulindac (*Clinoril*) and naproxen (*Naprosyn*), also **act by inhibiting cyclooxygenase. The side effects are less pronounced** than with aspirin.

  1. All produce some **GI bleeding.**

  2. **Renal toxicity** may occur, as a reduction of prostaglandins in the kidney reduces renal blood flow and renal function. The resulting salt and water retention can reduce the effectiveness of most antihypertensives.

  3. **Hepatitis** can also be induced.

D. Selective inhibitors of the COX-2 enzyme, e.g., celecoxib (*Celebrex*) and rofecoxib (*Vioxx*) appear to have:

    1. Good antiinflammatory activity.

    2. **Low gastric irritation**

    3. No effect on platelet aggregation

E. The NSAIDs and COX-2 inhibitors will decrease the pain and inflammation from arthritis, and the decreased inflammation can slow the joint damage. The disease continues to progress, however.

F. **Cytotoxic drugs** act by suppressing the immune system.

    1. **Methotrexate** (*Rheumatrex*) is effective at such low dosages that little toxicity actually occurs.

    2. **Cyclophosphamide** (*Cytoxan*) has more **cytotoxic** effects, such as bone marrow depression.

G. **The glucocorticoids** are the most potent anti-inflammatory drugs.

    1. They have a fast onset of action.

    2. **Many side effects** occur with chronic glucocorticoid administration, **including adrenal suppression, ulcers, and osteoporosis.**

    3. **Alternate day therapy** may reduce the severity of these side effects.

    4. Injection into a joint induces long term effects on the joint with little systemic toxicity.

H. **Antirheumatic drugs** have **slow onsets** of action, taking months to induce an effect.

    1. They have **no analgesic activity,** thus they should initially be combined with NSAIDs.

    2. They **reduce the progression of joint erosion,** probably by reducing the phagocytosis and immune responses that are responsible for this autoimmune disease.
        a. **Gold compounds** can be administered intramuscularly [e.g., **aurothioglucose** (*Solganal*)] or orally [e.g., **auranofin** (*Ridaura*)].
        b. **Penicillamine** (*Cuprimine*), a chelator, can be given orally.
        c. **Hydroxychloroquine** (*Plaquenil*), an antimalarial, is given orally; but can induce a **retinopathy.**

I. **Etanercept** (*Enbrel*), **an inhibitor of tissue necrosis factor,** has been approved for the treatment of rheumatoid arthritis.

J. Other rheumatoid and arthritic conditions are treated with the same groups of drugs, although the specific regimens may vary. The exception is gout.

VII. DRUGS FOR GOUT

A. **A disorder of uric acid metabolism** leads to the **hyperuricemia and acute gouty arthritis** that is characteristic of gout.

B. Many drugs can **reduce the gouty arthritic inflammation** without changing uric acid metabolism or elimination.

    1. **Colchicine** may act by decreasing the release of chemotactic factors which attract leukocytes to the inflamed joints. This results in a reduction in the release of inflammatory mediators.

    a. It has no effect on other inflammatory disorders, making it **useful in the diagnosis** of gout.

    b. **An antimitotic** effect on the gastric mucosa frequently leads to a **bloody diarrhea.**

  2. **NSAIDs,** such as indomethacin (*Indocin*), are very effective and safer than colchicine.

  3. **Glucocorticoids** or adrenocorticotropic hormone (ACTH) will reduce the acute attack, but should not be used chronically due to their marked toxicity. Glucocorticoids can be given intra-articularly, if the arthritic pain is localized to one or a few joints.

C. **Aspirin is contraindicated** in patients with gout, because it can reduce the renal clearance of uric acid and thereby increase the hyperuricemia.

D. **The hyperuricemia** can be reduced by 2 classes of drugs.

  1. **Uricosuric drugs,** such as **probenecid** (*Benemid*) and **sulfinpyrazone** (*Anturane*), **compete with uric acid transport** (especially reabsorption) in the proximal tubule of the kidney.

    a. The elimination of uric acid in the urine is increased.

    b. **Renal calculi** from uric acid crystals may form, thus the patient should ingest lots of **fluids with bicarbonate.**

    c. The mobilization of uric acid from the body stores **may induce an acute arthritic attack,** thus the patient should also be given colchicine or indomethacin.

    d. It is **inappropriate** to use uricosuric drugs:

      (1) During an **acute arthritic attack**

      (2) In patients with **renal failure**

      (3) When the **body burden of uric acid is very high,** such as in patients

        (a) **With many tophi**

        (b) **With hematological disorders**

        (c) **During cancer chemotherapy**

  2. **Inhibitors of uric acid synthesis** will reduce the production of uric acid, and are useful in patients who produce excessive amounts of uric acid.

    a. **Allopurinol** (*Zyloprim*) **inhibits xanthine oxidase.** It is also metabolized by xanthine oxidase to an active product, alloxanthine.

      (1) The uric acid concentration in the urine is reduced.

      (2) The **xanthine and hypoxanthine** concentrations in the urine are increased.

        (a) Xanthine and hypoxanthine are **more water soluble** than uric acid.

        (b) There are **multiple substances** in the urine, thus more total product can be excreted without causing crystalluria.

    b. The levels of 5-phosphoribosylpyrophosphate (PRPP), a precursor of purine synthesis, are also reduced by allopurinol.

    c. An acute attack can be induced, thus colchicine or indomethacin should be used in combination with the synthesis inhibitor.

VIII. DRUGS FOR ACNE

A. **Benzoyl peroxide** is a keratolytic that reduces acne.

B. Long-term treatment with **erythromycin or tetracyclines** is also effective.

C. **Isotretinoin** (*Accutane*), a vitamin A derivative, is administered orally for treatment of very severe cases of acne.

1. It inhibits the sebaceous glands.

2. The **side effects** can be very marked.
   a. It is **teratogenic.**
   b. **Hypervitaminosis A** can lead to irritated skin.

IX. VITAMINS

A. **Water-soluble vitamins are readily eliminated** by the kidney and are usually non-toxic.

B. **Fat-soluble vitamins can accumulate** and be more toxic, thus caution should be used if high doses are administered.

C. The deficiency and overdose syndromes for the vitamins are listed in Table 6–2.

D. The primary medical **uses** of vitamins are:

1. Treatment of **vitamin deficiencies**

2. **Prophylaxis** to avoid deficiencies in:
   a. Growing children
   b. Pregnant women
   c. Nursing mothers
   d. People on unusual diets

Table 6–2
Deficiency and Toxic States for Vitamins

	Deficiency state	Toxic state
Water soluble vitamins:		
Thiamine (B_1)	Berberi (alcoholism)	
Riboflavin (B_2)	Infrequent	
Niacin (nicotinic acid, B_3)	Pellagra	↓ serum triglycerides and cholesterol
		Flushing and GI distress
Pyridoxine (B_6)	Infrequent (isoniazid)	Peripheral neuropathy ↓ Anticonvulsant and L-dopa effects
Cyanocobalamin (B_{12})	Pernicious anemia	
Folic acid	Anemia Birth defects (anticonvulsants)	
Pantothenic acid	Infrequent	
Ascorbic acid (C)	Scurvy	
Biotin	Infrequent	
Fat soluble vitamins:		
Vitamin A	↓ Dark adaptation Night blindness	Dry, scaly skin
Vitamin D	Rickets	Hypercalcemia
Vitamin E	Infrequent	
Vitamin K	↓ Blood coagulation	Jaundice in newborn ↓ Effect of oral anticoagulants

Drugs in parentheses can induce the deficiency states.
↑ = increased; ↓ = decreased

7

Endocrine Pharmacology

I. PITUITARY HORMONES

A. The release of **growth hormone** from the pituitary gland is regulated in an inhibitory fashion by the hypothalamic hormone somatostatin.

    1. Challenge tests are available to:

        a. Increase the release of growth hormone, including:

            (1) Insulin, which induces hypoglycemia

            (2) Bromocriptine

            (3) L-Dopa

        b. Decrease the release of growth hormone, including:

            (1) Glucose

            (2) Glucocorticoids, which induce hyperglycemia

            (3) Somatostatin

    2. **A growth hormone deficiency before puberty** will result in pituitary **dwarfism.**

        a. **Somatrem** (*Protropin*) and **somatropin** (*Humatrope*) are human growth hormone produced by recombinant DNA technology.

            (1) Replacement therapy will increase growth.

            (2) Replacement therapy is ineffective after epiphyseal closure has occurred in the long bones.

        b. **Androgens and estrogens** also increase growth; however, they are less effective than growth hormone, and can induce epiphyseal closure which limits further growth.

    3. **Excessive growth hormone** leads to **gigantism** before puberty and **acromegaly** after puberty.

        a. **Surgical removal** of part of the pituitary gland is the treatment of choice.

        b. **Bromocriptine** (*Parlodel*), a dopamine receptor agonist, inhibits growth hormone release in patients with excessive growth hormone. This is the opposite of the effect seen in normal subjects.

        c. **Octreotide** (*Sandostatin*), a somatostatin analogue, will also inhibit growth hormone release.

B. Deficiencies of **other important anterior pituitary hormones** can also lead to clinical symptoms.

    1. Challenge tests are available for these hormones.

        a. **Gonadotropin releasing hormone** (GnRH) should increase the serum levels of follicle stimulating hormone (FSH) and luteinizing hormone (LH).

        b. **Corticotropin releasing hormone** (CRH) should increase the serum levels of adrenal corticotropic hormone (ACTH).

    c. Thyrotropin releasing hormone (TRH) should increase the serum levels of thyroid stimulating hormone (TSH).

  2. The **end-organ hormones,** rather than the deficient pituitary hormones, **are used** for replacement therapy of a pituitary deficiency.

  3. The **glucocorticoids should be replaced before the thyroid hormones** to avoid adrenal insufficiency.

C. Vasopressin [antidiuretic hormone (ADH)], released from the **posterior pituitary,** is an important regulator of urine osmolarity as it increases the permeability of the collecting ducts in the kidney to water. An inadequate vasopressin effect leads to **diabetes insipidus.**

  1. Diagnosis of the cause of the diabetes insipidus is based on the administration of vasopressin.

    a. If there is a **pituitary deficiency** of vasopressin, administered vasopressin will increase urine osmolarity.

    b. If the diabetes is **nephrogenic** in nature, administered vasopressin will have no effect on urine osmolarity.

  2. The treatment depends on the cause.

    a. If the diabetes insipidus is due to a **pituitary deficiency,** replacement therapy is instituted.

      (1) Vasopressin (*Pitressin*) can be given intramuscularly, but it can increase blood pressure.

      (2) Lypressin (*Diapid*), **administered intranasally,** has a duration of four hours.

      (3) Desmopressin (*DDAVP, Stimate*), administered intranasally, has a duration of **12 hours** and **does not increase blood pressure.**

    b. If the diabetes is **nephrogenic,** the **thiazides** (unexpectedly) are effective treatment.

D. Oxytocin (*Pitocin, Syntocinon*) is a posterior pituitary hormone that can be used to **increase uterine contractility.**

  1. Estrogens increase and progestins decrease the effects of oxytocin on the uterus.

  2. As term approaches, the number of oxytocin receptors in the uterine muscle increases; thereby increasing the sensitivity to oxytocin.

  3. The primary use for oxytocin is to induce labor at term.

    a. Low doses will increase the rhythmic contractions.

    b. High doses should be avoided because they can induce a sustained uterine contraction, leading to complications.

  4. Ergonovine (*Ergotrate*) also has oxytocic activity, however it induces a **sustained uterine contraction.** It is useful during the third stage of labor to:

    a. Induce expulsion of the placenta

    b. Reduce postpartum hemorrhaging by compressing the uterine blood vessels

  5. Premature labor can be reduced by administering a **β_2-adrenoceptor agonist,** such as ritodrine (*Yutopar*).

II. ADRENOCORTICAL STEROIDS

A. Cortisol, also called hydrocortisone, is the primary adrenal glucocorticosteroid.

  1. Transcortin [corticosteroid-binding globulin, (CBG)] binds 75% of the cortisol in the circulation.

    a. Bound hormone is inactive.

    b. **Estrogens and thyroxine increase CBG,** but do not change the free cortisol concentration.

    c. **Androgens decrease CBG.**

  2. Cortisol is metabolized by mixed function oxidases (MFOs) in the liver.

B. **The steroids diffuse** across the cell membranes and **bind to steroid receptors** in the cytoplasm. The steroid-receptor complex **migrates to the nucleus** and acts on DNA to **increase mRNA and protein synthesis.**

C. Three types of effects can be induced by these steroids.

  1. **Glucocorticoid effects** result from:

    a. **Enhanced gluconeogenesis** that leads to increased glucose production (diabetogenic) and increased glycogen synthesis and storage in the liver

    b. **Enhanced lipolytic effects** that redistribute fat

  2. **Mineralocorticoid effects** result from increased sodium ion exchange for potassium and hydrogen ions in the kidney.

    a. Hypokalemic alkalosis can be induced.

    b. The increased sodium load can lead to edema and hypertension.

  3. **Anti-inflammatory effects** occur, although the mechanism is not well established.

  4. The mineralocorticoid effects have been separated from the glucocorticoid and anti-inflammatory effects (Table 7–1); however, it has not been possible to separate the glucocorticoid actions from the anti-inflammatory actions

    a. Dexamethasone is the most selective for glucocorticoid activity.

    b. Fludrocortisone is the most selective for mineralocorticoid activity.

D. There are **many side effects** that can occur with the adrenocorticoids, including:

  1. **Hypokalemic alkalosis**

  2. **Glycosuria,** which can aggravate diabetes mellitus

  3. **Increased susceptibility to infections**

  4. **Myopathy**

  5. **Osteoporosis**

  6. **Symptoms of Cushing's syndrome**

  7. **Psychological effects**

  8. **ACTH suppression,** which induces adrenal atrophy from which recovery takes

Table 7–1

Relative Mineralocorticoid to Glucocorticoid Activities of the Adrenocortical Steroids, As Compared to Cortisol (hydrocortisone)

Adrenocortical Steroid	Mineralocorticoid activity / Glucocorticoid activity
Cortisol [(hydrocortisone) (*Cortef, Cortril*)]	1
Cortisone (*Cortone*)	1
Prednisone (*Deltasone*)	0.1
Dexamethasone (*Decadron, Hexadrol*)	0.01
Fludrocortisone (*Florinef*)	10

several months. Thus withdrawal from long-term glucocorticoid treatment should be slow and tapered.

E. Several drugs can **inhibit adrenal** cortical function.

   1. Aminoglutethimide (*Cytadren*) inhibits desmolase and reduces the production of all adrenal steroids.

   2. Metyrapone (*Metopirone*) reduces cortisol synthesis by inhibiting 11β-hydroxylase.

   3. Ketoconazole (*Nizoral*), an antifungal drug, reduces cortisol synthesis and release.

   4. Spironolactone (*Aldactone*) inhibits aldosterone receptors.

F. There are many **clinical uses** for the adrenal steroids.

   1. Adrenal insufficiency (Addison's disease) is treated with a glucocorticoid.
      a. Two thirds of the dose is administered in the morning to mimic the physiological levels.
      b. A mineralocorticoid is added if the insufficiency is primary (adrenal), but is usually not necessary for a secondary insufficiency (pituitary).
      c. For acute adrenal insufficiency, an intravenous glucocorticoid and saline are administered.

   2. Congenital adrenal hyperplasia is due to an enzyme deficiency (e.g., 21-hydroxylase), which leads to increased ACTH release. It is treated with a glucocorticoid and a mineralocorticoid is added, if needed.

   3. Dexamethasone is very useful in the **diagnosis** of Cushing's syndrome.

   4. The **anti-inflammatory effects** of the adrenal steroids are very useful in the treatment of **allergic reactions, inflammatory diseases, tissue rejection, and leukemias.**
      a. They are safe during short-term therapy.
      b. Many side effects occur with long-term therapy.
         (1) It is possible to reduce the pituitary suppression, somewhat, by using **alternate-day therapy.** This involves doubling the dose one day and using only NSAIDs on the next day.
         (2) Adrenocortical steroids should be used for chronic therapy only as a last resort.

III. FEMALE SEX HORMONES

A. Sex hormone binding globulin binds estradiol and testosterone.

B. Effects of estrogens include:

   1. Control of reproductive organs

   2. Control of sex characteristics

   3. Anabolic effects that promote growth, which are less than with androgens

C. The **estrogen preparations** are:

   1. Estradiol (*Estrace*), which is usually conjugated (*Premarin*) for a longer duration of action.

   2. Ethinyl estradiol (*Estinyl*)

   3. Mestranol

   4. Diethylstilbestrol (*Stilphostrol*), which is **non-steroidal**

D. Effects of the progestins include:

   1. Induction of the **secretory changes in the endometrium of the uterus** that are necessary for pregnancy

2. Induction of **menstruation,** when the progestin levels fall.

E. The **progestin preparations** include:

1. Progesterone, which is not useful due to a very short half-life

2. Medroxyprogesterone (*Provera*)

3. Norethindrone (*Norlutin*), which has some androgenic activity

4. Levonorgestrel (*Norplant*)

5. Desogestrel, a newer preparation

F. **Side effects** have been ascribed mostly to the estrogens.

1. Some have **minor** consequences, such as
  a. **Nausea and vomiting**
  b. **Edema**
  c. **Breast tenderness**

2. Some have **major** consequences, such as
  a. **Thrombophlebitis, deep vein thrombosis, and pulmonary embolism,** especially in smokers older than 35 years of age. The increased risk is similar to the risk during pregnancy.
  b. **Breast cancer** (controversial) and **endometrial cancer**
  c. Fluid retention and mild hypertension

G. Drugs which activate MFOs, e.g., rifampin, can reduce the effectiveness of the estrogen-progestin contraceptives.

H. There are many **uses** for the female sex steroids.

1. **Contraceptives** can act by many different mechanisms.
  a. **The combined oral estrogen-progestin** (from days 5 to 25) **reduces FSH and LH release** by the negative feedback inhibitory action of the estrogen on the pituitary, and this reduces ovulation.
    (1) The new preparations have lower estrogen concentrations to reduce the side effects.
    (2) Phasic preparations have more progestin during the later phases of the menstrual cycle.
  b. **The continuous oral progestins (minipills)** reduce implantation of the fertilized ovum. A common side effect is irregular menstruation.
  c. **Depot medroxyprogesterone** (*Depo-Provera*) or **levonorgestrel** (*Norplant*) are progestins that are useful when compliance is a concern.
  d. **Acute, high-dose estrogen therapy** is used, postcoitally, to reduce implantation.
  e. **Mifepristone (RU 486) is an anti-progesterone** substance that blocks the preparation of the uterus for pregnancy. It is usually combined with prostaglandins when used to induce abortions.
  f. **Nonoxynol-9** acts as a spermicide.
  g. The sequential estrogen (days 5 to 25) and progestin (days 20 to 25) oral contraceptives were withdrawn from the market because they induce endometrial cancer.

2. **Hypogonadism** is treated by replacement therapy with physiological doses of sex steroids. This includes:
  a. **Menopausal symptoms** induced by the loss of female sex hormones.
    (1) **Estrogens will decrease the symptoms of menopause.**
    (2) **Progestins** are usually added to the regimen to reduce the high incidence of **endometrial cancer** when estrogens are used alone.

b. Amenorrhea

(1) Estrogen–progestin preparations will **induce menstruation.**

(2) **Growth and sexual development** will be induced when the sex hormones are administered at the age of puberty.

c. Dysfunctional uterine bleeding

3. Inhibition of ovarian function can be induced by pharmacological doses of sex steroids.

a. Dysmenorrhea is reduced, due to the inhibition of ovulation. Indomethacin is also effective because it inhibits prostaglandin release, which may be involved in inducing the dysmenorrhea.

b. Hirsutism due to ovarian androgens is reduced.

c. Some cancers are treatable with sex hormones or sex hormone antagonists.

I. An inappropriate indication for estrogens is a threatened miscarriage. If used in such a manner, estrogens can induce **vaginal adenomas in female offspring after puberty,** and may also affect male offspring. Estrogens are now **contraindicated during pregnancy.**

IV. FERTILITY DRUGS

A. Clomiphene (*Clomid*) is an **antiestrogen that reduces the feedback inhibition** of estrogen on the pituitary gland and hypothalamus.

1. Increased release of FSH and LH **enhances ovulation.**

2. A functional pituitary gland and functional ovaries are required.

3. The incidence of multiple pregnancies is increased.

B. Human menopausal gonadotropins (hMG) (*Pergonal*) and **human chorionic gonadotropins** (hCG) (*Follutein, Pregnyl*) have **FSH and LH activities;** thus a functional pituitary gland is not required. Follitropin β (*Follistim*) is a recombinant FSH with similar properties.

C. GnRH preparations act on the pituitary gland.

1. Pulsatile administration of **gonadorelin** (*Factrel*) induces the release of FSH and LH.

2. Sustained administration of **leuprolide** (*Lupron*) decreases the release of FSH and LH, which is useful in the **treatment of infertility from endometriosis.**

D. Danazol (*Danocrine*) is a testosterone derivative that reduces gonadotropin release.

1. Endometrial atrophy is produced, which reduces **endometriosis.**

2. Upon discontinuing the danazol, fertility is increased.

E. Bromocriptine (*Parlodel*) is a **dopamine receptor agonist** that reduces prolactin release from the pituitary gland. It increases fertility in patients with **hyperprolactinemia.**

V. MALE SEX HORMONES

A. These sex hormones have **androgenic and anabolic** activities.

B. Many **preparations** are available.

1. Testosterone is usually administered, **intramuscularly,** as an ester (*Delatestryl*) to prolong the duration of action.

2. Methyltestosterone (*Metandren, Testred*) and **fluoxymesterone** (*Halotestin*) are effective when given **orally** and have longer durations of action than testosterone.

3. Nandrolone (*Durabolin*) is an **anabolic** steroid, although it still has some androgenic effects.

C. The **side effects** include:

1. Masculinization

2. Edema

D. The **uses** for the male sex hormones include:

1. Treatment of hypogonadism
   a. Potency and fertility (if given with gonadotropins) are increased.
   b. Growth is increased, although epiphyseal closure induced by the steroids can limit further growth.

2. Treatment of cryptorchism, for which **hCG** is used

3. Treatment of prostate cancer, for which leuprolide (*Lupron*) is used

4. Anabolic actions
   a. To hasten recovery after an injury
   b. To treat anemias

E. An inappropriate use of the steroids is to increase athletic performance. The anabolic steroids can cause:

1. Reduced growth, after an initial growth spurt, by inducing premature epiphyseal closure in young athletes

2. Reduced fertility due to feedback inhibition by the steroids on gonadotropin release

3. Virilization in females

4. Hepatotoxicity and hepatic tumors

5. Edema and hypertension

F. Spironolactone (*Aldactone*) and **flutamide** (*Eulexin*) have **antiandrogen activity** and can be used to treat hirsutism, prostate cancer, and precocious puberty.

VI. THYROID HORMONES

A. The thyroid preparations include:

1. Levothyroxine (T_4) (*Levothroid, Synthroid*), which is a pure chemical
   a. It is **highly bound** to thyroxine binding globulin **(TBG).**
   b. The half-life is **7 days.**

2. Liothyronine (**L-triiodothyronine, T_3**) (*Cytomel*), which is also a pure chemical
   a. It is less well bound than T_4 to TBG, thus it is **more potent.**
   b. The half-life is **1 day,** which is much shorter than the half-life of T_4.

3. Desiccated thyroid, which is powdered animal thyroid glands

4. Thyroglobulin (*Proloid*), which is extracted from animal thyroids

5. Liotrix, which is a combination of T_4 and T_3

6. TSH (*Thytropar*) and **TRH (protirelin)** (*Thypinone*), which are used for diagnostic purposes

B. Hypothyroidism, whether primary, secondary, or tertiary in nature, is the major indication for the thyroid hormone preparations.

  1. T_4 is usually preferred, and treatment is initiated slowly to avoid cardiovascular symptoms.

  2. T_4 will reduce the symptoms of hypothyroidism and reduce TSH release which reduces the goiter.

  3. T_3 has too rapid an onset, and is only preferred for the treatment of hypothyroid coma.

  4. Side effects from hormone replacement are due to an **increase in metabolic rate** and include:
  a. Flushing
  b. Weight loss
  c. Increased appetite
  d. Tachycardia
  e. Angina

  5. In the hypothyroid newborn, aggressive treatment within one month of birth is necessary to avoid cretinism. After 3–4 months of untreated hypothyroidism in the newborn, brain dysfunction will occur.

C. Antithyroid drugs act by several different mechanisms.

  1. The thioamides, such as **propylthiouracil and methimazole** (*Tapazole*) inhibit thyroid hormone synthesis.
  a. Reduced I_2 binding to tyrosine and reduced coupling of iodotyrosines leads to a depletion of thyroid hormones.
    (1) The release of T_4 and T_3 is reduced.
    (2) Increased TSH release from reduced feedback inhibition can induce a **goiter.**
    (3) The onset is very **slow** because the large stores of hormones have to be depleted.
  b. Propylthiouracil also inhibits the peripheral conversion of T_4 to T_3.

  2. Iodide in large amounts rapidly reduces thyroid hormone release, although the effect is transient. It also reduces the vascularity of the thyroid gland.

  3. Radioactive iodine (^{131}I) is concentrated in the thyroid, where β-irradiation can destroy some of the thyroid cells.

  4. Thiocyanate and perchlorate block the iodide concentrating mechanism in the thyroid. They are not used, however, because aplastic anemia can be induced.

  5. The sympathetic blockers [e.g., propranolol (*Inderal*)] do not affect the thyroid, but do rapidly **reduce the myocardial stimulation** that occurs with elevated thyroid hormone levels.

D. Hyperthyroidism can be treated in three ways.

  1. Administration of **thioamides** will reduce the synthesis and release of thyroid hormones.
  a. Since a goiter can occur if the patient becomes hypothyroid, T_4 may be added to the regimen to reduce TSH release.
  b. This is not a permanent cure.
  c. Propylthiouracil and methimazole do cross the placenta and will affect the fetus.

2. **A partial thyroidectomy** can result in a permanent cure.

    a. Possible adverse consequences of surgery are hypoparathyroidism and **hypothyroidism.**

    b. Propylthiouracil or iodide are used pre-operatively to reduce the size and vascularity of the thyroid gland.

3. ^{131}I, given orally, will destroy some of the thyroid cells. ^{131}I treatment:

    a. Has a **slow onset,** thus treatment with antithyroid drugs may be necessary until ^{131}I becomes effective.

    b. Can result in **hypothyroidism**

    c. **Must be avoided during pregnancy**

    d. Could theoretically induce genetic abnormalities (but probably doesn't)

E. **Thyroid storm** (acute hyperthyroid crisis) can be treated with **propranolol and antithyroid drugs.**

F. **Thyroid cancer** can be treated with ^{131}I, if the cancer cells concentrate iodide.

VII. HORMONES AFFECTING CALCIUM METABOLISM

A. Three hormones are involved in the regulation of the serum calcium concentration (Figure 7–1).

    1. **Parathyroid hormone** release, induced by hypocalcemia, increases serum calcium by increasing the:

        a. **Formation of active 1,25 dihydroxyvitamin D$_3$** in the kidney, which increases the **absorption of calcium in the gut**

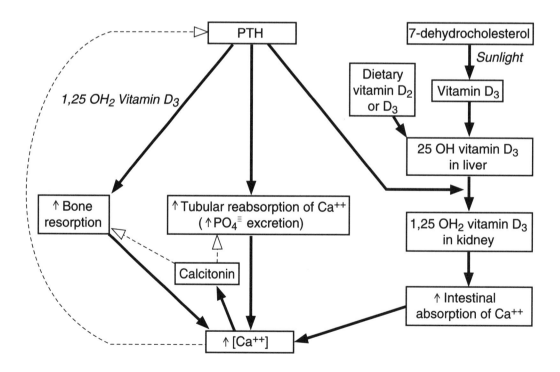

Figure 7–1. Regulation of calcium metabolism by parathyroid hormone, vitamin D and calcitonin. Ca^{++} = calcium; OH=hydroxy; OH_2=dihydroxy; $PO_4^{\equiv}$=phosphate; PTH=parathyroid hormone

  b. Bone resorption of calcium
  c. Kidney reabsorption of calcium (and increasing phosphate excretion)

2. Vitamin D₃ from the diet or from exposure to sunlight is hydroxylated to **25 hydroxyvitamin D₃, calcifediol** (*Calderol*), in the liver.
  a. This intermediate is further hydroxylated in the kidney to **1,25 dihydroxyvitamin D₃, calcitriol** (*Rocaltrol*).
  b. Dihydroxyvitamin D₃ **increases the intestinal absorption of calcium.**

3. Calcitonin release, in response to hypercalcemia, decreases bone resorption.

B. Hypoparathyroidism results in hypocalcemia, hyperphosphatemia and increased membrane excitability (hypocalcemic tetany).

  1. Treatment involves the administration of a **vitamin D preparation and calcium.** Parathyroid hormone is not very useful as it must be given intramuscularly.

  2. Calcitriol is preferred for acute treatment.

  3. Pseudohypoparathyroidism can be treated with high doses of vitamin D, which appear to directly increase bone resorption.

C. Osteomalacia (hypovitaminosis D) is also treated with a **vitamin D preparation.**

  1. If GI absorption is poor, vitamin D can be administered parenterally.

  2. If liver function is reduced, calcifediol or calcitriol can be administered.

  3. If kidney function is reduced, calcitriol or **dihydrotachysterol** (*Hytakerol*) can be administered.
  a. Dihydrotachysterol has a **rapid onset.**
  b. It is metabolized in the **liver** to the active form.

D. Hyperparathyroidism results in **hypercalcemia.**

  1. Surgery is the preferred mode of treatment.

  2. Corticosteroids can be used to **reduce the absorption of calcium** by the intestine.

  3. Acute treatment involves the administration of:
  a. Fluids
  b. Loop diuretics, which increase calcium excretion by the kidneys
  c. Phosphate, if hypophosphatemia is present

E. Hypervitaminosis D results in hypercalcemia and is acutely treated much like hyperparathyroidism.

F. Osteoporosis is a skeletal disorder in which calcium hormone function is normal.

  1. Treatment of postmenopausal osteoporosis involves the administration of:
  a. Vitamin D
  b. Calcium
  c. Estrogen receptor modulators, such as raloxifene (*Evista*), which
    (1) Stimulates bone and lowers serum lipids.
    (2) Has no effect on the endometrium or breasts.

  2. Other treatment modalities can be used.
  a. Calcitonin can be administered, intranasally.
  b. Alendronate (*Fosamax*) is a bisphosphonate that stabilizes bone.

G. Paget's disease involves a rapid turnover of the calcium in bone. **Treatment** utilizes:

  1. Calcitonin (*Calcimar*), parenterally. Salmon calcitonin is the most active form.

2. **Etidronate** (*Didronel*) or alendronate, which are bisphosphonates that reduce bone turnover. They are **effective when given orally** and have the same efficacy as calcitonin.

VIII. DRUGS FOR DIABETES MELLITUS

A. Diabetes is due to an inadequate effect of insulin that can lead to **hyperglycemia, ketonemia,** and **ketoacidosis.**

B. Type 1 (insulin-dependent) diabetes mellitus results from the loss of endogenous insulin, while type 2 (non-insulin-dependent) diabetes mellitus is probably due to insulin resistance often associated with obesity.

C. There are many **preparations** with hypoglycemic actions.

   1. **Insulin** is a **polypeptide** that is ineffective when given orally and is usually administered intramuscularly or subcutaneously.

      a. Insulin

         (1) increases glucose transport into muscle and adipose tissue.

         (2) increases glycogen synthesis, decreases glycogenolysis and decreases gluconeogenesis in liver tissue.

         (3) decreases lipolysis in adipose tissue

      b. Several sources are available.

         (1) **Bovine insulin** has three amino acids that are different from human insulin.

         (2) **Porcine insulin** has only one amino acid that is different from human insulin. It is available as a conventional or a purified (less antigenic) preparation.

         (3) **Human insulin** (*Humulin*) is produced by recombinant DNA technology.

      c. **Regular insulin (crystalline zinc insulin)** has a fast onset and is the only insulin preparation that can be given intravenously. It also has a short duration of action.

      d. Insulin is conjugated with proteins or crystallized in various forms which slows the onset and increases the duration of action. **NPH** and **lente insulins** with durations up to 24 hours are the most useful.

      e. **Lispro insulin** (*Humalog*) is a new rapid acting, short duration preparation.

   2. **Oral antidiabetic drugs** are also effective.

      a. **The sulfonylureas increase the insulin release** from the pancreas, and enhance the peripheral effectiveness of insulin, thus a functional pancreas is required.

         (1) **Tolbutamide** (*Orinase*) is short acting and is metabolized in the liver by oxidation.

         (2) **Chlorpropamide** (*Diabinese*) is long acting and is partially excreted in the unchanged form by the kidney.

         (3) **Glyburide** (*DiaBeta, Micronase*) and **glipizide** (*Glucotrol*) are second generation sulfonylureas.

      b. **Metformin** (*Glucophage*) is a biguanide that **enhances the hepatic response** to insulin. A rare, but serious, complication is lactic acidosis.

      c. **Acarbose** (*Precose*) is an **α-glucosidase inhibitor** which slows the breakdown of carbohydrates in the gut. It has gastrointestinal side effects.

      d. **Rosiglitazone** (*Avandia*) **reduces insulin resistance** in type 2 diabetes mellitus. Liver function should be monitored in patients on this drug.

D. The **side effects** of insulin and the sulfonylureas can be very severe.

   1. **Hypoglycemia** can occur from excessive doses, inadequate food intake, exercise, or alcohol.

   a. **CNS effects,** which can progress to convulsions, lead to a **sympathetic activation** (e.g., tachycardia). Propranolol will block this sympathetic activation making it more difficult for diabetics to sense that they are hypoglycemic.

   b. The hypoglycemia can be **reversed by:**

   (1) Ingestion of candy, orange juice, or other **sugar** source
   (2) Glucagon, intramuscularly or subcutaneously
   (3) Glucose, intravenously

   2. **Insulin antibodies** can lead to **cutaneous allergic reactions or resistance** to insulin. The risk of antibody formation for the insulin preparations is: bovine > porcine > purified porcine > human.

   3. Increases in body weight frequently occur.

E. **Treatment** of diabetes involves **balancing of caloric intake, exercise, and hypoglycemic medications.**

   1. The diet is a major factor in diabetic control, and the caloric intake should be constant and regular.

   2. Patients with **type 1** diabetes mellitus must use **insulin.**

   3. Patients with **type 2** diabetes mellitus can use either **insulin** or **oral hypoglycemic drugs.** Insulin is preferred for type 2 diabetes mellitus in patients with:

   a. Reduced renal function
   b. Reduced hepatic function
   c. Gestational diabetes
   d. Persistent hyperglycemia
   e. Cardiovascular risk factors

   4. The efficacy of treatment should be followed by **self-monitoring of blood glucose** by the patient and physician monitoring of glycosylated hemoglobin.

   5. Effective treatment should **nearly eliminate the acute symptoms** of diabetes, including the hyperglycemia, polyphagia, polydipsia, polyuria, hypoglycemia, and ketoacidosis.

   6. Based on clinical studies, **rigid control** of blood glucose **probably also reduces the chronic complications** of diabetes, including:

   a. Neuropathy
   b. Retinopathy
   c. Nephropathy
   d. Cardiovascular disease

F. **Diabetic ketoacidosis or hyperosmolar (non-ketotic) coma** should be managed with:

   1. **Fluid and electrolytes, especially potassium**

   2. Crystalline zinc insulin, intravenously

   3. Correction of acidosis

   4. Carbohydrates

IX. DRUGS FOR HYPOGLYCEMIA

A. **Glucagon,** which is physiologically released from alpha cells in the pancreas, **increases glycogenolysis and gluconeogenesis.**

    1. These actions **increase the blood glucose** concentration in diabetics who are hypoglycemic.

    2. The effectiveness will be lost when the **glycogen stores are depleted.**

    3. It is a polypeptide that must be given **parenterally.**

B. **Glucose** can be administered orally or parenterally to treat hypoglycemia in diabetics.

C. **Diazoxide** (*Proglycem*) is an antihypertensive, when given intravenously.

    1. After **oral** administration, it **reduces insulin release** from the pancreas; thus it is ineffective for the treatment of insulin-induced hypoglycemia.

    2. It is useful to treat the hypoglycemia from a **hyperinsulinoma.**

D. Many hormones can increase the serum glucose concentration, including:

    1. Glucocorticoids

    2. Growth hormone

    3. Epinephrine

    4. Estrogens and progestins

    5. Thyroid hormone

8

Drugs for Bacterial Infections

I. PRINCIPLES OF BACTERIAL CHEMOTHERAPY

A. Bacterial chemotherapy involves the administration of drugs that **kill or slow the growth of bacteria without affecting host cells.** This phenomena is called **selective toxicity.**

B. **Bactericidal drugs kill bacteria,** often by inhibiting cell wall synthesis.

   1. Bactericidal drugs include
      a. β-Lactams
         (1) Penicillins
         (2) Cephalosporins
         (3) Aztreonam
         (4) Imipenem
      b. Aminoglycosides
      c. Quinolones
      d. Vancomycin

   2. Bactericidal drugs are necessary for
      a. Patients with severe infections
      b. Patients with severe or debilitating diseases
      c. Patients who are immunocompromised

C. **Bacteriostatic drugs** only **inhibit replication of bacteria,** often by reducing protein synthesis.

   1. The immune system eradicates the infection.

   2. Bacteriostatic drugs include:
      a. Tetracyclines
      b. Erythromycin
      c. Chloramphenicol
      d. Clindamycin
      e. Sulfonamides
      f. Trimethoprim

D. **Single drugs are preferred** to treat infectious diseases, unless a drug combination is the accepted mode of therapy (usually to reduce the development of resistance). Inappropriate drug combinations can:

   1. Increase the incidence of side effects

   2. Result in antagonism between drugs

   3. Increase the risk of superinfections

E. Bacterial resistance to drugs can be

1. **Natural** (e.g., no target site in the bacteria)

2. **Acquired**

   a. Resistance acquired by **mutation** is unusual, although it is common with tuberculosis (TB) because there is a large population of bacteria (See XV "Drugs for Tuberculosis").

   b. Resistance acquired by **R-factors** on plasmids is a common, **very rapid** method of acquiring resistance that often involves resistance to many antibiotics.

F. Changes of the bacterial flora in the gastrointestinal tract that are induced by antibiotics frequently lead to symptoms of GI irritation, such as nausea, vomiting, and diarrhea.

G. Superinfections due to an **overgrowth of insensitive indigenous microbes,** such as *Pseudomonas, Clostridium,* and *Candida,* are most prevalent

1. With broad-spectrum antibiotics

2. With long-term therapy

3. In patients with severe illnesses

Table 8-1
Overview of Antibacterial Drugs*

Class	Site of Action	Activity	Admini- stration	Clearance	Distribution to CSF	Toxicity	Spectrum	Acquired Resistance
Penicillin G	W	C	O,P	K	s	H,G	+,N	E,A,R
Penicillins, extended	W	C	O,P	K	s	H,G,N	+,~	E,A,R
Cephalosporins, 1st	W	C	o,P	K	s	H	+,~,N	E,A,R
Cephalosporins, 3rd	W	C	o,P	K	G	H,S	+,−,N	E,A,R
Aztreonam	W	C	P	K	s	G	−	E
Imipenim/Cilastatin	W	C	P	K	i	G,H,C	+,−,N	R
Aminoglycosides	30S	C	P	K	i	O,K	−	E,R
Tetracyclines	30S	S	O,p	K,L	s	B,P,S	+,−,N	R
Erythromycin	50S	S	O,p	L	i	G,L	+,N	A,R
Chloramphenicol	50S	S	O,P	L	G	A	+,−,N	E
Clindamycin	50S	S	O,P	L	i	G,S	+,N	A,R
Vancomycin	W	C	P	K	s	N,O,K	+	A
Quinolones	G	C	O,P	K,L	G	G,E	+,−	A,R
Sulfonamides	FA	S	O	L,K	G	A,H,U	+,−,N	A,R
Trimethoprim	FA	S	O	K	G	A	+,−,N	A
Metronidazole	D	C	O,P	L	G	D	N	

*There are many exceptions to the general properties listed in this table.
Site of Action: W, cell wall; 30S, ribosome; 50S, ribosome; G, gyrase; FA, folic acid metabolism; D, DNA
Activity: C, bactericidal; S, bacteriostatic
Administration: O, oral; o, ocasionally oral; P, parenteral; p, ocasionally parenteral
Clearance: K, kidney; L, liver
Distribution to CSF: G, good; s, some; i, inadequate
Toxicity: A, anemias; B, binds calcium; C, convulsions; D, disulfiram-like; E, erosion of cartilage; G, gastrointestinal; H, hypersensitivity; K, kidney toxicity; L, liver toxicity; N, non-allergic rash; O, ototoxic; P, photosensitivity; S, superinfection; U, crystalluria
Spectrum: +, gram(+); −, gram(−); ~, some gram(−); N, anaerobes
Acquired Resistance: A, active site change; E, enzymatic break-down; R, reduced accumulation

H. The properties of the antibacterial drugs are summarized in Table 8–1.

II. PENICILLINS

A. The **active nucleus** of the penicillin molecule is a 4-membered ring, called the **β–lactam ring** (Figure 8–1).

B. Penicillin binds to **penicillin binding proteins** and induces many effects that inhibit cell wall synthesis (e.g., **inhibition of transpeptidases**).

   1. **Cross-linking of the bacterial cell wall is reduced.**

   2. The cell wall is weakened and the bacteria rupture due to the high internal osmotic pressure, thus the penicillins are **bactericidal.**

C. The **pharmacokinetics** of penicillin G affect how it is used.

   1. It is relatively **unstable in acid,** thus the bioavailability is low. It can be administered orally, however, the serum penicillin concentrations are variable after this route of administration.

   2. There is **poor penetration into the cerebrospinal fluid (CSF),** unless inflammation is present.

   3. **Active renal tubular secretion** results in a short half-life. Probenecid, which blocks the active secretion, will reduce the renal clearance of penicillin G.

   4. Penicillin G procaine, intramuscularly, and penicillin G benzathine, intramuscularly, have long durations of action due to slow absorption from the site of injection.

D. Although the penicillins are very safe antibiotics, they have some important **adverse effects.**

   1. **Hypersensitivity** reactions can develop.

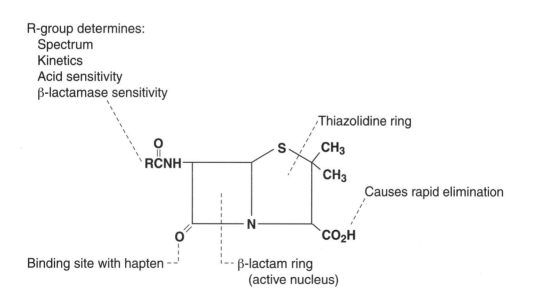

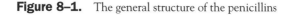

Figure 8–1. The general structure of the penicillins

    a. Immediate hypersensitivity reactions, characterized by **anaphylaxis,** occur within 20 minutes.

       (1) Penicillin interacts with proteins to form **minor determinants** which act as haptens for inducing the immediate hypersensitivity reaction.

       (2) The reaction is mediated by **IgE antibodies.**

       (3) Anaphylactic reactions should be treated with **epinephrine.**

    b. Accelerated (occurring within 1 day) and **delayed** (occurring within 1 week) reactions are less severe, often leading to skin rashes.

       (1) Penicilloic acid, which is a product of the breakdown of penicillins, interacts with proteins to form the **major determinants,** which act as haptens for inducing the reactions.

       (2) These reactions are mediated by **IgG or IgM antibodies.**

    c. Patients may display hypersensitivity to the first dose. This hypersensitivity is probably due to the environmental levels (e.g., in food) of penicillins.

    d. Cross-sensitivity between the penicillins is very high.

    e. Skin tests are available to check for hypersensitivity.

       (1) Penicillin G is useful, but somewhat unreliable.

       (2) Penicilloyl-polylysine is a major determinant.

       (3) Minor determinants are not widely available.

2. Superinfections can develop, especially with the broad-spectrum penicillins, such as ampicillin.

3. Sodium loading from the penicillins is most common with carbenicillin and ticarcillin, which are disodium salts.

4. Convulsions, caused by γ-aminobutyric acid (GABA) receptor blockade, can be induced at high dosages of penicillins.

5. Non-allergic skin rashes can occur with ampicillin, especially in patients with infectious mononucleosis.

E. The **spectrum** of penicillin G includes:

1. Gram-positive bacteria

2. Gram-negative cocci, but not most other gram-negative bacteria

3. Some anaerobes

F. Penicillin G is especially effective for treating infectious diseases due to:

1. *Neisseria meningitidis*

2. Streptococci

3. *Clostridium perfringens*

4. *Fusobacterium*

5. *Treponema pallidum*

G. Acquired **resistance** to penicillin G is usually due to **penicillinases or β-lactamases,** which split the active part of the molecule, the β-lactam ring.

H. Amidases are used to alter the side chain of penicillin G (Table 8–2), resulting in groups of:

1. Natural penicillins. Penicillin V is more effective after oral administration than penicillin G.

2. Penicillinase-resistant penicillins. These penicillins are useful for the treatment of infections involving penicillinase-producing bacteria, such as *Staphylococcus aureus* or *epidermidis.*

3. **Extended-spectrum penicillins.** These penicillins have more gram-negative activity than penicillin G.

a. Ampicillin or amoxicillin are useful for infectious diseases due to:

(1) *Enterococcus faecalis*

(2) *Proteus mirabilis*

(3) *Listeria monocytogenes*

b. The antipseudomonal penicillins have higher activity versus *Pseudomonas aeruginosa.*

c. All extended-spectrum penicillins are penicillinase-sensitive.

(1) Either **clavulanic acid** or **sulbactam,** which are **β-lactamase inhibitors,** can be combined with the extended-spectrum penicillins.

(2) Resistant organisms will be more sensitive to this combination.

III. CEPHALOSPORINS

A. The structure of the cephalosporins (Figure 8–2), with a β-lactam ring and a dihydrothiazine ring, is very similar to that of the penicillins; and the pharmacological **properties** are also similar to those of the penicillins.

1. **Inhibition of transpeptidases** leads to an inhibition of cell wall synthesis resulting in a **bactericidal** effect.

2. Most cephalosporins are eliminated by active tubular secretion in the kidney.

3. Penetration into the CSF is poor, unless inflammation is present.

4. The **side effects** are also similar to those from the penicillins, including

Table 8–2
Properties of the Penicillins

	Effectiveness when taken orally	Resistance to penicillinases	Spectrum
Natural penicillins			
Penicillin G	Variable	None	Narrow
Penicillin V (*Pen-Vee, V-Cillin*)	Good	None	Narrow
Penicillinase-resistant penicillins			
Methicillin (*Staphcillin*) (side effect: nephritis)	Poor	Yes	Narrow
Cloxacillin (*Tegopen, Cloxapen*)	Good	Yes	Narrow
Nafcillin (*Unipen*)	Variable	Yes	Narrow
Dicloxacillin (*Dynapen*)	Good	Yes	Narrow
Extended-spectrum penicillins			
Ampicillin (*Omnipen*) (side effect: non-allergic rash)	Good	None	Extended
Amoxicillin (*Amoxil, Larotid*)	Better	None	Extended
Extended-spectrum antipseudomonal penicillins			
Carbenicillin (*Geocillin*)	Poor	None	Extended
Ticarcillin (*Ticar*)	Poor	None	Extended
Piperacillin (*Pipracil*)	Poor	None	Extended

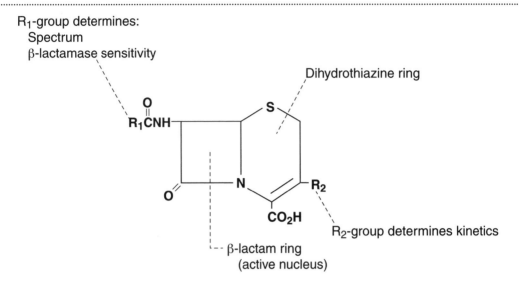

R$_1$-group determines:
  Spectrum
  β-lactamase sensitivity

Dihydrothiazine ring

R$_2$-group determines kinetics

β-lactam ring
(active nucleus)

Figure 8–2.   The general structure of the cephalosporins

    a. Hypersensitivity
       (1) There is **some cross-hypersensitivity with the penicillins.**
       (2) In patients with a history of a mild accelerated or mild delayed reaction to a penicillin, the cephalosporins may be considered.
       (3) In patients with a history of an immediate reaction to a penicillin, the cephalosporins should be avoided.
    b. **Superinfections,** especially with the broader spectrum cephalosporins.
    c. Nephrotoxicity

B. The cephalosporins also have important **differences from the penicillins.**

    1. The anti-bacterial **spectrum is broader.**

    2. They are **more resistant to β-lactamases.**

    3. Most are ineffective when taken orally, due to break-down by acid in the stomach.

C. Four generations of cephalosporins are available.

    1. **First-generation** cephalosporins include cefazolin (*Ancef,Kefzol*) and oral cepha-lexin (*Keflex*).
       a. These have **narrow spectrums for cephalosporins,** but the spectrums are sim-ilar to ampicillin.
       b. They have some resistance to β-lactamases.
       c. They are the **most active** cephalosporins **for gram-positive bacterial infec-tions.**

    2. **Second-generation** cephalosporins include cefoxitin (*Mefoxin*), oral cefuroxime (*Zinacef*), and oral cefaclor (*Ceclor*). They have broader spectrums and more resis-tance to β-lactamases.

    3. An important use of first and second-generation cephalosporins is **prophylaxis during surgery** if an infection is likely to occur.

    4. As a group, the **third-generation** cephalosporins have:

a. The **broadest spectrums**
b. The **highest activities against gram-negative bacteria**
c. The **lowest activities against gram-positive bacteria**
d. The **highest resistance to β-lactamases**
e. The **highest lipid solubilities**
f. The **best penetration into the CSF**
g. The most clinical usefulness, including treatment of infectious diseases due to:
    (1) *Neisseria gonorrhoeae*
    (2) *Escherichia coli*
    (3) *Haemophilus ducreyi*
    (4) *Haemophilus influenzae*, if severe
    (5) *Klebsiella pneumoniae*
    (6) *Proteus*, indole positive
    (7) *Salmonella*

5. There are also some unique properties of **individual third-generation cephalosporins.**
    a. **Ceftriaxone** (*Rocephin*) has the **longest half-life** (8 hours) of any cephalosporin.
    b. **Cefixime** (*Suprax*) is an **oral** preparation.
    c. **Ceftazidime** (*Fortaz*) is the best **anti-pseudomonal** cephalosporin.
    d. **Cefoperazone** (*Cefobid*) is eliminated **(70%) in the bile,** and is thus very useful in patients with renal failure.

6. Cefepime (*Maxipime*) is a fourth generation cephalosporin.

IV. OTHER β-LACTAMS

A. **Aztreonam** (*Azactam*) is a **monobactam.**

    1. It decreases cell wall formation, and thus is **bactericidal.**

    2. **Only aerobic gram-negative bacteria,** especially *Pseudomonas*, are affected. There is no activity against gram-positive bacteria or anaerobes.

    3. It is resistant to most β-lactamases.

    4. The kinetics are similar to the penicillins, although it must be **administered parenterally.**

B. **Imipenem with cilastatin** (*Primaxin*) inhibits cell wall transpeptidation.

    1. This results in **bactericidal** activity against most bacteria, thus imipenem has a **very broad spectrum.**

    2. It is resistant to most β-lactamases.

    3. It **distributes to most tissues** in the body, except the cerebral spinal fluid.

    4. Imipenem is **nephrotoxic.**
        a. Metabolism of imipenem in the kidney by **dehydropeptidases** leads to an inactive product that is nephrotoxic.
        b. **Cilastatin inhibits the dehydropeptidases** and eliminates the nephrotoxicity, thus it is always administered in combination with imipenem.

    5. It is especially useful for treating infectious diseases due to:
        a. *Campylobacter fetus*
        b. *Serratia*

V. AMINOGLYCOSIDES AND SPECTINOMYCIN

A. The **aminoglycosides** include **gentamicin** (*Garamycin*), **tobramycin** (*Nebcin*), **amikacin** (*Amikin*), neomycin (*Mycifradin*) and streptomycin.

1. **Inhibition of protein synthesis** occurs as a result of **irreversible** aminoglycoside binding to the **30S ribosomal subunit.**
a. An inactive initiation complex is formed.
b. Misreading of the mRNA template occurs.

2. Although aminoglycosides act as protein synthesis inhibitors, they are **bactericidal.** This may be due to the irreversible binding at the site of action.

3. The **selective toxicity** may relate to the fact that **humans do not have the 30S ribosomal subunits.**
a. Mammals have 80S ribosomes composed of 60S and 40S subunits.
b. Bacteria have 70S ribosomes composed of 50S and 30S subunits.

4. Aminoglycosides are only active against **gram-negative bacteria** that are **aerobes,** because the drugs must be accumulated in the bacteria by active transport, which is oxygen-dependent. The activity is maintained even after the plasma drug concentration falls. This is called a **post-antibiotic effect.**

5. The **pharmacokinetics** are typical for large, polar molecules.
a. **Parenteral administration** is necessary.
b. Distribution is limited to the extracellular fluid.
c. They **do not reach the CSF.**
d. **Elimination** occurs via **glomerular filtration,** thus the creatinine clearance is used to determine the maintenance dose.

6. **Resistance** is mediated by **R-factors** transmitted by conjugation.
a. Bacterial **enzymes** can inactivate the aminoglycosides.
b. Membrane uptake of the aminoglycosides can be reduced.
c. Amikacin induces a much lower incidence of microbial resistance than the other aminoglycosides.

7. The aminoglycosides are **very toxic,** thus it is important to **monitor the serum concentrations** of these drugs.
a. **Ototoxicity** can lead to:
(1) Loss of equilibrium
(2) Loss of hearing
b. **Nephrotoxicity** can occur.
c. **Neuromuscular blockade** can reduce respiratory function, especially after surgery.

8. They are very useful to treat infectious diseases due to:
a. *Enterococcus faecalis*, if severe
b. *Pseudomonas aeruginosa*

9. An aminoglycoside in combination with a β-lactam provides broad (empiric) antibiotic treatment.

B. Spectinomycin (*Trobicin*) also **inhibits protein synthesis** by binding the **30S** ribosomal subunit.

1. It is only **bacteriostatic.**

2. The only important indication is as an alternate treatment for **gonorrhea.**

VI. TETRACYCLINES

A. This class of antibiotics includes **tetracycline** (*Achromycin, Panmycin*) and **doxycycline** (*Vibramycin*), which are **bacteriostatic inhibitors of protein synthesis.**

    1. Reversible binding to the **30S ribosomal subunit** inhibits the acceptor (A) site on the mRNA.

    2. Binding of tRNA to the mRNA-ribosomal complex is blocked.

B. **Selective toxicity** occurs because the tetracyclines are **actively accumulated by bacteria,** but not actively accumulated by host cells.

C. **Resistance** is mediated by **R-factors** that **reduce the active drug accumulation.**

D. The **pharmacokinetics** vary depending on the specific drug.

    1. All tetracyclines can be administered orally.

        a. Tetracycline, in particular, is **chelated and inactivated by calcium (milk), magnesium, aluminum (antacids) and iron,** and should be taken when the stomach is empty.

        b. Doxycycline is less avidly chelated and can be taken with a meal.

    2. Some tetracyclines are cleared by metabolism in the liver and some are cleared by glomerular filtration in the kidney.

    3. **Doxycycline,** uniquely, is cleared as a **chelate in the feces.** The elimination is not dependent on either liver or kidney function.

E. The **spectrum is very broad,** and the tetracyclines are especially useful for infectious diseases involving

    1. *Chlamydia*

    2. *Rickettsia*

    3. *Mycoplasma pneumoniae*

    4. *Borrelia burgdorferi*

F. These antibiotics have few **side effects.**

    1. **Do not administer tetracyclines to children** because chelation of calcium
        a. Can **discolor developing teeth**
        b. Can **reduce growth** in developing bone

    2. **Photosensitivity** can occur.

    3. Hepatotoxicity and nephrotoxicity have been reported.

    4. As they have broad spectrums, **superinfections** from *Clostridium* and *Candida* can develop.

VII. ERYTHROMYCIN

A. This **macrolide** antibiotic is a **bacteriostatic** inhibitor of protein synthesis. Reversible binding to the **50S ribosomal subunit** of gram-positive microorganisms inhibits translocation of the peptidyl molecule from the A-site to the P-site on the mRNA.

B. It is effective when taken orally and is **eliminated in the bile** in the unaltered form.

C. **Reduction of mixed function oxidase (MFO) activity** enhances the effects of many drugs metabolized by MFOs (e.g., theophylline).

D. The spectrum includes **gram-positive and intracellular bacteria.**

    1. Erythromycin (*Ilosone, Erythrocin*) is especially useful for infectious diseases involving:
        a. *Chlamydia*
        b. *Mycoplasma pneumoniae*

        c. *Legionella pneumophila*

      2. It is also a useful alternative to the penicillins for gram-positive infections.

   E. **Cholestatic hepatitis** and gastrointestinal side effects can occur

   F. New macrolides are very useful.

      1. **Clarithromycin** (*Biaxin*) is **more stable in acid** than erythromycin.

      2. **Azithromycin** (*Zithromax*) has a **long half-life** (3 days).

VIII. CHLORAMPHENICOL

   A. **Bacteriostatic inhibition of protein synthesis** results from reversible binding of chloramphenicol (*Chloromycetin*) to the **50S** ribosomal subunit.

      1. This decreases the binding of tRNA to the A–site.

      2. As a result, protein elongation is reduced.

   B. It is effective when **given orally, penetrates membranes very well,** and **readily reaches the CSF.**

   C. **Metabolism** by glucuronyl transferase **(glucuronide conjugation)** occurs in the liver.

   D. **Toxicity** is a major limitation with chloramphenicol.

      1. A **gray baby syndrome** can be induced when chloramphenicol is administered to newborns. **Slow metabolism,** which is due to a lack of glucuronyl transferase, results in toxic blood concentrations of chloramphenicol when standard doses are administered.

      2. **Anemias** can be induced.

         a. **Dose-dependent bone marrow depression** results from inhibition of mitochondrial 70S ribosomes.

         b. An infrequent, **irreversible aplastic anemia** that is **not dose-related** and is **frequently fatal** has limited the usefulness of chloramphenicol to seriously ill patients who cannot be treated with safer drugs.

   E. The **spectrum** of activity is **very broad, including anaerobes,** but it is only used as an alternative drug to treat infections, such as *Salmonella typhi* and *Haemophilus influenzae*. It is bactericidal for *H. influenzae*.

   F. **Resistance** occurs due to **R-factors** that code for the enzyme, chloramphenicol **acetyltransferase,** which acetylates and inactivates the drug.

IX. CLINDAMYCIN

   A. **Bacteriostatic inhibition of protein synthesis** results from binding of clindamycin (*Cleocin*) to the **50S** ribosomal subunit.

   B. Clindamycin is effective when given **orally** and is useful to treat **anaerobic infections.**

   C. The incidence of **pseudomembranous colitis** (a superinfection from *Clostridium difficile*) is high and this limits the usefulness of clindamycin. This superinfection should be **treated with metronidazole** or vancomycin, given orally.

X. VANCOMYCIN

   A. **Binding of vancomycin** (*Vancocin*) **to cell wall precursors** leads to an **inhibition of cell wall synthesis** that is **bactericidal.**

B. Because it is poorly absorbed by the oral route, vancomycin is given **intravenously** except when being used to treat enteric infections.

C. It is cleared by renal **glomerular filtration.**

D. The high activity of vancomycin against **gram-positive microorganisms** makes it useful as the last alternative to treat **methicillin-resistant *Staphylococcus aureus*** or *epidermidis* and penicillin-resistant *Streptococcus pneumoniae*.

E. **Side effects** include:

1. Ototoxicity

2. Nephrotoxicity

3. Erythema ("red neck syndrome"), due to histamine release

XI. STREPTOGRANINS

A. **Quinupristin/dalfopristin** (*Synecid*) is a new drug combination that **inhibits protein synthesis** by an action at the 50S ribosomal subunit.

B. It has bactericidal activity and can be **used to treat vancomycin-resistant infections.**

XII. QUINOLONES

A. **Norfloxacin** (*Noroxin*) and **ciprofloxacin** (*Cipro*) inhibit bacterial **DNA gyrases,** which results in a **bactericidal** effect. They are structurally similar to nalidixic acid, a urinary tract antiseptic.

B. **Resistance** develops due to a mutational **change in the gyrase.**

C. The **spectrum** is **very broad,** although there is **no effect on anaerobes.** Ciprofloxacin is very useful for treatment of:

1. Infections due to *Shigella*

2. Urinary tract infections due to *Pseudomonas aeruginosa*

D. Both oral and intravenous administration are effective, and the drugs distribute widely in the body.

E. **Elimination** is primarily due to **renal secretion** of the active drug.

F. Erosion of cartilage by the quinolones can lead to tendinitis and tendon rupture.

XIII. SULFONAMIDES AND TRIMETHOPRIM

A. The sulfonamides [e.g., sulfisoxazole (*Gantrisin*)] are **analogues of para-aminobenzoic acid (PABA)** that compete with PABA in the synthesis of folic acid (Figure 8–3).

1. The **decrease of tetrahydrofolic acid** inhibits DNA synthesis, primarily by decreasing thymidylate synthesis.

2. **Selective toxicity** occurs because:
a. **Bacteria have no active transport for folate and must synthesize it.** This synthesis is blocked by the sulfonamides.
b. **Humans cannot synthesize folate.** They must obtain it from the diet and it is actively transported into the host cells. Inhibition of folate synthesis has no host effects.

3. These drugs are usually **bacteriostatic;** although with the selective absence of thymine, they can be bactericidal.

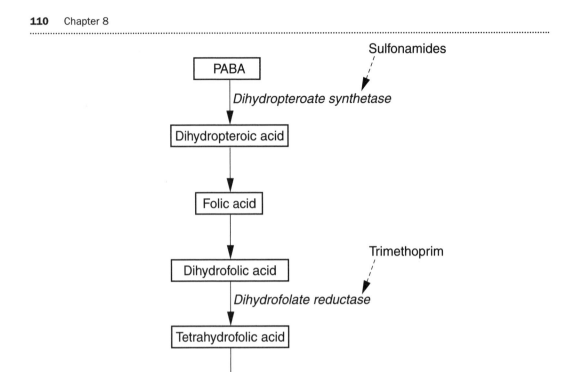

Figure 8–3.   The synthesis of folic acid. The sites of sulfonamide and trimethoprim actions are indicated. PABA=para-aminobenzoic acid

    4. The **spectrum is very broad** and they **distribute to all body fluids.**

    5. The major limitation of the sulfonamides is the **R–factor mediated resistance** which is very common.

    6. **Side effects** can usually be avoided.
        a. **Displacement of bilirubin** from plasma albumin binding sites can induce **ker‐nicterus** in the newborn.
        b. Due to their poor solubility, some of the older sulfonamides can **crystallize in the urine.**
        c. **Hypersensitivity reactions** (e.g., Stevens-Johnson syndrome) do occur, par‐ticularly with the long-acting sulfonamides which are now rarely used.
        d. **Hemolytic anemia** can be induced.

    7. The important **indications** for use of the sulfonamides are:
        a. **Urinary tract infections** that are acute and uncomplicated
        b. **Recurrent otitis media**

  B. **Trimethoprim** (*Proloprim, Trimpex*) is a **competitive inhibitor of dihydrofolate re‐ductase.**

    1. This inhibitory action leads to effects on folic acid synthesis that are similar to the sulfonamides, although the onset is more rapid.

2. **Selective toxicity** occurs because the **bacterial reductase is 20,000 times as sensitive** as the human reductase.

C. **Trimethoprim** and the **sulfonamides** (e.g., sulfamethoxazole) are usually combined (*Bactrim, Septra*).

    1. A **synergistic** effect occurs with the combination because 2 steps in folic acid synthesis are inhibited.

    2. This is a very useful combination for treating:
        a. **Recurrent urinary tract infections**
        b. **Chronic prostatitis**
        c. **Nocardiosis**
        d. *Pneumocystis carinii*
        e. **Upper respiratory tract infections** from *Haemophilus influenzae*

    3. The combination can induce a **folate deficiency in the host,** leading to an **anemia** that is treatable with folinic acid.

XIV. MISCELLANEOUS ANTIMICROBIALS

A. **Urinary tract antiseptics are rapidly eliminated in the active form by the kidney,** so the drug concentrations in the urine are very high. This makes them useful for treating urinary tract infections.

    1. **Nitrofurantoin** (*Macrodantin*) damages DNA and has a **broad antimicrobial spectrum.**

    2. **Methenamine** (*Mandelamine*) is broken down by the **low pH** of urine to **formaldehyde,** which is bactericidal, especially against **gram-negative bacteria.**

B. **Bacitracin** (*Baciguent*) inhibits cell wall synthesis by **decreasing precursor transport** to the cell wall.

C. **Polymixin B** and **colistin** (*Coly-Mycin*) **increase membrane permeability,** leading to the loss of essential intracellular substances.

XV. DRUGS FOR TUBERCULOSIS

A. **Drug combinations,** often initially with 4 drugs, are always used in the long–term treatment (9–12 months) of TB to **avoid the development of antibiotic resistance.** Single drug therapy is only useful for preventive purposes.

B. **Isoniazid** (*Nydrazid*) decreases the **synthesis of mycolic acid,** which is a cell wall component in the *Mycobacterium*.

    1. It is **bactericidal,** although resistance develops rapidly by mutation due to the large population of bacteria in an active infection.

    2. Oral administration of isoniazid is effective and the drug **distributes to all body fluids** and to all sites of infection.

    3. **Clearance** from the body involves **acetylation** in the liver, the rate of which has a **genetic** variation.
        a. **Fast acetylators will have lower blood concentrations.**
        b. **Slow acetylators are more likely to develop toxicity.**

    4. **Side effects** from isoniazid include:
        a. **Hepatitis,** which increases in incidence with **age** and use of alcohol.
        b. **Peripheral neuritis** due to increased pyridoxine excretion. This can be avoided by giving **pyridoxine.**

C. **Rifampin** (*Rifadin, Rimactane*) inhibits the β-subunit of DNA-dependent RNA **poly-merase,** which reduces RNA synthesis in the bacteria.

   1. Rifampin is also **bactericidal** for *Mycobacterium* and has **good penetration** into tissues and tuberculous lesions.

   2. It is also used **prophylactically** for patients exposed to:
      a. *Neisseria meningitidis*
      b. *Haemophilus influenzae,* **type b**

   3. **Metabolism** occurs in the liver and it activates MFOs.

   4. **Side effects** include:
      a. **Hepatotoxicity**
      b. **Orange coloring of tears, sweat, and urine**
      c. **A flu-like syndrome**

D. **Pyrazinamide** is **bactericidal** and effective when given orally.

E. **Ethambutol** (*Myambutol*) inhibits mycolic acid synthesis, but is only **bacteriostatic.** It can also **impair red–green vision.**

F. **Streptomycin** is **bactericidal,** but it

   1. must be administered **parenterally**

   2. does not penetrate into cells

   3. **does not distribute** as widely in the body as the other drugs.

G. Treatment of **leprosy** (*Mycobacterium leprae*) involves long term administration of drug combinations of:

   1. **Sulfones [e.g., dapsone** (*Alvosulfon*)] which are PABA analogues that reduce folic acid synthesis.

   2. Rifampin

   3. Thalidomide (*Thalomid*)

9

Drugs for Infections from Eukaryotic Organisms and Viruses

I. ANTIFUNGAL DRUGS

A. **Amphotericin B** (*Fungizone*) **binds ergosterol** in fungal cells and **increases the membrane permeability** by forming membrane pores.

   1. Amphotericin B is **fungicidal** at high dosages.
      a. It is the drug of choice for most systemic fungal infections.
      b. It has no antibacterial activity.

   2. Selective toxicity occurs because there is less binding to cholesterol in host cell membranes.

   3. **Slow parenteral** administration is necessary.

   4. The **side effects** are **very severe,** including:
      a. A febrile response
      b. A delayed nephrotoxicity

   5. Amphotericin B lipid complex (*Abelcet Injection*) has similar effects, but less toxicity.

B. **Flucytosine** (*Ancobon*) is metabolized by deaminases in the fungal cells to the active substance, **fluorouracil.**

   1. Fluorouracil inhibits fungal DNA and RNA synthesis.

   2. An advantage of flucytosine is **wide distribution,** even to the CNS.

C. The **azoles** interfere with **ergosterol synthesis,** thereby increasing fungal membrane permeability.

   1. They are only **fungistatic.**

   2. They are valuable alternatives to amphotericin because of their effectiveness when administered orally and mild side effects.

   3. **Ketoconazole** (*Nizoral*)
      a. can only be administered orally
      b. **is poorly absorbed if gastric pH is high** (e.g., with antacids)
      c. has some **hepatoxicity**
      d. **inhibits MFO,** which will slow the metabolism of many drugs. Cortisol and testosterone synthesis will also be reduced.

   4. **Fluconazole** (*Diflucan*) and **itraconazole** (*Sporonex*) have properties that are similar to ketoconazole, except:

      a. Intestinal absorption of these drugs is **not affected by changes of gastric pH**

      b. They can be given orally or **intravenously.**

      c. Fluconazole penetrates much better into the CSF.

E. Nystatin (*Nilstat, Mycostatin*) acts like amphotericin B in that it binds ergosterol; however, it is only used **topically.**

F. Griseofulvin (*Gris-PEG, Grisactin*) **binds to keratin** and is used orally for fungal infections of the skin, hair, and nails.

    1. Disruption of mitotic spindles, which decreases mitosis, leads to a fungistatic action.

    2. Griseofulvin has a **very low water solubility.**

      a. The duration of action is very long (months) after oral administration.

      b. It undergoes metabolism in the liver and activates the MFOs.

II. ANTIPROTOZOAL DRUGS

A. Malaria is a common protozoal disease in tropical climates.

    1. Blood schizonticidal drugs clear the *Plasmodium* from the erythrocytes.

      a. Chloroquine (*Aralen*) is selectively **concentrated** ($100\times$) by red blood cells that are infected with the parasites.

        (1) It acts on all erythrocytic *Plasmodium* infections, **except chloroquine-resistant** *Plasmodium falciparum*, now very prevalent, and **chloroquine-resistant** *Plasmodium vivax.*

        (2) Once a week, oral administration is effective because chloroquine is highly concentrated in the liver and has a long half-life.

      b. Pyrimethamine (*Daraprim*) **inhibits dihydrofolate reductase,** leading to reduced folic acid synthesis, especially in parasites.

        (1) It is often combined with a sulfonamide [(e.g., sulfadoxine (*Fansidar*)].

        (2) Teratogenicity has been reported in animals.

      c. Quinine has a **very rapid onset** and short duration, making it useful for treating a **severe acute attack. Side effects** are:

        (1) Cinchonism

        (2) Arrhythmias

      d. Mefloquine (*Lariam*) is a quinine derivative that has a **long half-life** and can be administered orally.

      e. Tetracyclines also have antimalarial activity.

    2. Primaquine is the only drug which can eliminate the tissue forms of the parasites.

      a. It is active on the **exoerythrocytic forms** and the gametes of *Plasmodium vivax* and *Plasmodium ovale.*

      b. Hemolytic anemia can occur in patients with a glucose-6-P-dehydrogenase deficiency.

    3. Prophylaxis is usually provided for travelers to countries where malaria is endemic. **Mefloquine** (1 dose/week) is given from 1 week before the trip to 4 weeks after.

B. Amebiasis involves both gastrointestinal and tissue sites.

    1. Metronidazole (*Flagyl*) acts on *Entamoeba histolytica* in the intestinal and hepatic sites, but does not eliminate the intestinal cysts.

      a. It is metabolized by microorganisms to the active form which **targets DNA in anaerobes,** such as *Entamoeba, Gardnerella, Bacteroides,* and *Clostridium.*

      b. A **disulfiram-like** reaction can occur, if alcohol is ingested.

    2. Iodoquinol (*Yodoxin*) is an **intestinal amebicide** that is not absorbed, thus there are no systemic effects or side effects.

C. Other infections respond to drug therapy.

    1. *Toxoplasma gondii* infections are treated with pyrimethamine and a sulfonamide.

    2. *Pneumocystis carinii* infections are treated with trimethoprim and sulfamethoxazole.

    3. Metronidazole is useful to treat infections from:
      a. *Trichomonas vaginalis*
      b. *Giardia lamblia*

III. ANTHELMINTICS

A. Anthelmintics are used to treat parasitic worm infections due to nematodes, cestodes, or trematodes.

B. The specific treatment of a nematode infection will depend on the type of nematode involved.

    1. Intestinal nematodes (*Enterobius*, *Ascaris*, *Trichuris*, *Necator*, and *Ancylostoma*) are the easiest to treat because the drugs do not have to be absorbed into the body of the host.

      a. Pyrantel (*Antiminth*) **activates nicotinic cholinoceptors** inducing a **muscle paralysis** in the helminth.

      b. Mebendazole (*Vermox*) **and albendazole** (*Zentel*) **inhibit glucose uptake.**

      c. The weakened parasites are then eliminated in the feces.

    2. Tissue nematodes can be divided into 2 types.

      a. Filarial nematodes include *Wuchereria*, *Brugia*, *Onchocerca*, *Loa*, and *Dipetalonema*.

        (1) Diethylcarbamazine (*Hetrazan*) may increase the helminth susceptibility to the host **immune system.**

          (a) It is **most active against the microfilaria** and least active against the adult filaria.

          (b) An allergic reaction can result from the parasitic break-down products.

        (2) Ivermectin (*Mectizan*) **opens GABA-sensitive chloride channels** which induces a muscle paralysis.

      b. Non-filarial tissue nematodes include *Angiostrongylus* and *Trichinella*.

        (1) Thiabendazole (*Mintezol*) **inhibits fumarate reductase,** which is unique to helminths.

        (2) Mebendazole (*Vermox*) and **albendazole** (*Zentel*) are also effective.

C. Cestode infections (*Taenia saginata*, *Taenia solium*, *Diphyllobothrium latum* and *Hymenolepis nana*) can be treated with **praziquantel** (*Biltricide*).

    1. Muscle stimulation and paralysis are induced in the helminths.

    2. Vacuolization of the cuticle also occurs.

    3. The tissue forms of *T. solium* (cysticercosis) are also effectively treated with either praziquantel or albendazole.

D. Trematode infections, such as schistosomiasis, can be treated with **praziquantel** (*Biltricide*).

IV. ANTIVIRAL DRUGS

A. Amantadine (*Symmetrel*) and **rimantadine** (*Flumadine*) act on RNA viruses by **inhibiting the uncoating** of viral nucleic acids, which reduces viral replication.

1. These drugs are used primarily for the **prophylaxis** of **type A influenza viral infections.**

2. **Treatment** with either of these drugs is effective if initiated **within 48 hours** after the initial appearance of symptoms.

B. Oseltamivir (*Tamiflu*) is effective prophylactically for **both type A and type B influenza viral infections**

C. Acyclovir (*Zovirax*) is a guanine analogue that is a relatively safe antiviral drug.

    1. It is safe because it has **2 sites** of selective toxicity (Figure 9–1).
        a. **Only viruses can phosphorylate acyclovir to acyclovir monophosphate.**
        b. **Acyclovir triphosphate is more active on viral DNA polymerases.**

    2. The clinical **indications** include:
        a. **Genital and labial herpes simplex virus (HSV) types 1 or 2. There is no effect on the latent forms.**
        b. **Herpes encephalitis and keratitis**
        c. **Varicella-zoster virus**

D. Ganciclovir (*Cytovene*) is an analogue of acyclovir that is used for **cytomegalovirus (CMV) and Epstein-Barr virus** infections.

E. Foscarnet (*Foscavir*) is an alternate drug for the treatment of **mucocutaneous HSV and CMV.**

F. Ribavirin (*Virazole*) is used to treat the **respiratory syncytial virus and chronic hepatitis C.**

G. Zidovudine (*Retrovir*), formerly called azidothymidine (AZT), is a thymidine analogue that is converted to the triphosphate form, which is then incorporated into viral DNA and terminates viral DNA synthesis.

    1. Zidovudine **inhibits HIV reverse transcriptase.**

    2. It is used:
        a. In the treatment of **HIV-positive and AIDS patients.**
        b. In pregnant women with HIV to reduce the transmission of HIV to the newborn

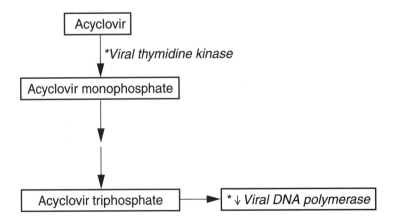

Figure 9–1. Mechanisms of selective toxicity (*) for acyclovir.

    c. To reduce the incidence of HIV in health-care workers exposed to the virus, e.g. needlestick

    3. Bone marrow depression may occur.

H. Didanosine (*Videx*) is another reverse transcriptase inhibitor that is used in HIV patients.

I. Ritonavir (*Norvir*) acts by **inhibiting proteases** that cleave viral protein precursors.

    1. It is used in combination with drugs like AZT and didanosine for the treatment of HIV.

    2. These regimens can dramatically reduce the symptoms of AIDS, however no regimen can eliminate HIV.

10

Cancer Chemotherapy

I. PRINCIPLES OF CANCER CHEMOTHERAPY

A. Most anticancer drugs **affect cell division.**

    1. They act preferentially on **rapidly proliferating cells.**

    2. Smaller tumors have a higher growth fraction.

        a. Consequently, they are more susceptible to the anticancer drugs.

        b. Adjuvant chemotherapy is used with surgery or radiation to treat undetectable metastases, when they are small and highly sensitive to anticancer drugs.

    3. Non-dividing cells **will survive** chemotherapy.

B. Some drugs are **cell cycle phase specific.**

    1. The cell cycle phases include:

        a. G_1, the phase after mitosis. Some G_1 cells can move into a resting, non-dividing state, G_0.

        b. S, the DNA synthesis phase

        c. G_2, the phase before mitosis

        d. M, the mitotic phase

    2. Methotrexate kills in **S-phase** (DNA synthesis phase).

    3. Vincristine and vinblastine kill in **M-phase** (mitotic phase).

C. Cells are killed in a first-order manner (a constant percentage is killed with each course of therapy).

D. Immunocompromised patients usually have poorer responses to anticancer treatment.

E. Combination therapy is common.

    1. Each drug in the combination should be **active** against the tumor.

    2. The drugs should have **different mechanisms** of action.

    3. The drugs should have **different toxicities.**

    4. The drugs are usually administered in treatment cycles and time must be allowed for host tissue recovery between cycles.

F. There are many **standard toxicities** that occur with most anticancer drugs.

    1. Myelosuppression is common because the bone marrow is a rapidly proliferating tissue.

        a. This is usually the dose-limiting side effect.

b. The leukopenia is greater than the thrombocytopenia, which is greater than the anemia.

c. The drugs for which bone marrow depression is not the dose–limiting toxicity include:
(1) Hormones
(2) Vincristine
(3) Bleomycin
(4) Asparaginase
(5) Cisplatin

2. Other rapidly proliferating cells that are affected include:
a. GI epithelium
b. Germinal epithelium
c. Hair follicles

3. Nausea and vomiting are common side effects that can be managed with anti-emetics, including:
a. Phenothiazines
b. Dronabinol (*Marinol*)
c. Metoclopramide (*Reglan*)
d. Ondansetron (*Zofran*), a 5-HT$_3$ antagonist
e. Glucocorticoids, such as dexamethasone

4. Tissue necrosis may occur at the site of injection.

5. Some anticancer drugs have **unique organ toxicities.**
a. Daunorubicin and doxorubicin are cardiotoxic.
b. Bleomycin induces pulmonary toxicity.
c. Vincristine is neurotoxic.
d. Cisplatin is nephrotoxic.

6. Mutagenicity, teratogenicity, and carcinogenicity can occur, especially with the alkylating agents.

7. A large cell kill can lead to **hyperuricemia** and crystalluria. These can be reduced with **allopurinol** (*Zyloprim*).

II. ANTICANCER DRUGS

A. Alkylating agents are usually cell cycle **phase non-specific.**

1. Nitrogen mustards form a very reactive **immonium** intermediate.
a. The intermediate attacks nucleophilic groups, especially **guanine,** leading to:
(1) Cross-linking of DNA
(2) Linking of bases in the same DNA strand
(3) Linking of bases to water or other molecules
b. Compounds with **2 reactive sites** have **greater activity.**
c. The cells will not replicate normally.
d. The cells can repair the DNA; thus, the mustards are **proliferation dependent** because rapidly dividing cells have less time to repair the DNA before DNA replication occurs.
e. Resistance occurs due to:
(1) Reduced drug uptake by the cancer cells
(2) Increased rate of DNA repair
f. Cross-resistance between alkylating agents is common.
g. Bone marrow depression is the dose-limiting side effect for these drugs.
h. The nitrogen mustards include:

    (1) Mechlorethamine (*Mustargen*), which is a potent **vesicant** with a **very short half-life** (a few minutes).

        (a) It reacts with tissues quickly, especially those near the site of injection.

        (b) **Phlebitis** occurs at the injection site.

    (2) Cyclophosphamide (*Cytoxan*), which is a **prodrug** that is metabolized to the active forms.

        (a) **Phosphoramide mustard** and acrolein are 2 active alkylating metabolites.

        (b) As the prodrug form is inactive, it can be given **orally** and it is not a vesicant.

        (c) The metabolites are eliminated in the urine which can irritate the bladder, leading to a **sterile hemorrhagic cystitis.**

    (3) Chlorambucil (*Leukeran*), which is effective after oral administration and is the slowest-acting and least toxic alkylating agent.

    (4) Melphalan (*Alkeran*)

2. The **nitrosoureas** include:

    a. **Lomustine** (*CCNU, CeeNu*) and **carmustine** (*BiCNU*), which are **highly lipophilic.**

        (1) They can **penetrate to the CSF.**

        (2) Unlike most other cytotoxic drugs, they are useful to treat CNS cancers or metastases in the CNS.

    b. **Streptozocin** (*Zanosar*), which accumulates in the **beta cells of the pancreas** and can produce **insulin shock,** an unusual side effect for an anticancer drug.

3. **Busulfan** (*Myleran*), **thiotepa** (*Thioplex*), and **dacarbazine** (*DTIC*) are other alkylating anticancer drugs.

4. **Cisplatin** (*Platinol*) and carboplatin (*Paraplatin*) are alkylating agents that bind to guanine in the DNA molecule.

    a. They are not phase-specific.

    b. **Nephrotoxicity** is the dose-limiting side effect.

B. **Antimetabolites** are usually **phase-specific, especially S-phase–specific.**

1. **Methotrexate** (*Folex*) is an analogue of folic acid which competitively inhibits the enzyme, **dihydrofolate reductase.**

    a. Tetrahydrofolate levels are decreased.

        (1) Decreased DNA, RNA, and protein synthesis occurs.

        (2) The primary effect is a decrease of **thymidylate synthesis.**

        (3) The highest activity occurs with low thymidine derivatives and normal RNA and normal proteins.

    b. It is S–phase specific and **self–limited** because it slows the movement of cells into the S–phase.

    c. Toxicity can be **reversed by leucovorin** (citrovorum factor) which is directly converted to tetrahydrofolate.

    d. Resistance can be due to:

        (1) Increased production of dihydrofolate reductase

        (2) Decreased affinity of the enzyme for methotrexate

        (3) Decreased active transport of methotrexate into the cancer cells

    e. Due to a low water solubility, **crystalluria and renal damage** can occur.

2. **Purine analogues** must be phosphorylated to be active.

    a. **Thioguanine** is converted to thioguanine monophosphate and deoxythioguanosine triphosphate, which is **incorporated into tumor cell DNA.**

(1) Thioguanine monophosphate also inhibits amidotransferases, which leads to reduced purine synthesis.

(2) It is S-phase specific.

b. Mercaptopurine (*Purinethol*) is converted to thioinosine monophosphate, which inhibits amidotransferase.

(1) It is **inactivated by xanthine oxidase.**

(2) As a result, **allopurinol** will decrease the metabolism and increase the toxicity of mercaptopurine.

3. Fluorouracil (*Efudex, Adrucil*) is an important **pyrimidine analogue.**

a. The phosphorylated form, fluorodeoxyuridine monophosphate, decreases the activity of thymidylate synthase.

b. This effect can be enhanced by leucovorin and reversed by thymidine.

C. Some **antibiotics** can be used as anticancer drugs.

1. **Dactinomycin** (*Cosmegen*), also called actinomycin D, **intercalates** between bases, especially guanine, in DNA.

a. This reduces DNA-dependent RNA polymerase activity, which reduces RNA synthesis.

b. It is cytotoxic at **all phases** of the cell cycle and is **not proliferation dependent.**

c. Resistance occurs due to decreased drug entry into the cells.

2. **Doxorubicin** (*Adriamycin*) and **daunorubicin** (*Cerubidine*) also **intercalate** into DNA, but there is **no base specificity.**

a. Resistance occurs due to decreased drug entry into the cells and there is cross-resistance between doxorubicin and daunorubicin, and often with dactinomycin.

b. A **cumulative cardiotoxicity** occurs due to **superoxide anion.**

3. Bleomycin (*Blenoxane*) induces **fragmentation of DNA.**

a. The effects of intercalating agents are enhanced.

b. **Delayed pulmonary toxicity** can be produced.

D. **Steroid hormones** can induce palliation of some cancers.

1. Their activity depends on the presence of the **steroid receptors** (e.g., estrogen receptors).

2. Hormone active substances include the antiestrogen tamoxifen (*Nolvadex*), estrogens, progestins, androgens, and corticosteroids.

E. There are several **inhibitors of chromosomal function.**

1. The vinca alkaloids, **vincristine** (*Oncovin*) and **vinblastine** (*Velban*), enhance the **depolymerization** of the **tubulin in the mitotic spindles,** thereby disrupting spindle function.

a. **Mitosis is inhibited (M-phase specific).**

b. Vinblastine displays standard toxicity, however **neurotoxicity is the dose-limiting side effect of vincristine.**

2. Etoposide (*VePesid*) **inhibits topoisomerases,** resulting in breaks of the DNA strands. Cells are arrested in late S- or G_2-phase.

3. Paclitaxel (*Taxol*) **enhances microtubule formation** and thereby affects cell division.

F. **Miscellaneous drugs** have unique actions.

1. **Asparaginase** (*Elspar*) metabolizes asparagine and glutamine.

      a. Tumors with no asparagine synthetase are sensitive to asparaginase, because any asparagine taken up by the tumors will be metabolized.

      b. It has none of the standard anticancer drug toxicities.

      c. **Hypersensitivity** reactions can occur due to the proteinaceous nature of this drug.

  2. Mitotane (*Lysodren*) induces an adrenocortical necrosis and is useful to treat adrenocortical cancers.

III. IMMUNOMODULATORS

  A. Immunosuppressants are used to suppress the rejection of transplanted organs.

    1. **Corticosteroids** act on many processes to suppress the immune response.

      a. They have **no cytotoxic activity.**

      b. **Anti-inflammatory** effects are very useful.

    2. **Cytotoxic drugs suppress the bone marrow,** and thereby reduce the immune reaction. They have **no anti-inflammatory effects.**

      a. **Azathioprine** (*Imuran*) is a **purine analogue** that is converted to mercaptopurine which reduces DNA synthesis.

        (1) It is **S-phase specific.**

        (2) The side effect profile is similar to the anticancer drugs.

      b. **Cyclophosphamide** (*Cytoxan, Neosar*) is a **phase non-specific** immunosuppressant.

      c. **Methotrexate** (*Folex*) is also useful.

    3. **Cyclosporine** (*Sandimmune*) is a **selective immunosuppressant.**

      a. **T-lymphocyte activation is reduced,** probably as a result of decreased interleukin release.

      b. B-lymphocyte and mature T-lymphocyte functions are not affected.

      c. There is **no myelosuppression.**

      d. **Nephrotoxicity** is the major complication.

  B. The immune potentiator, **levamisole** (*Ergamisol*), increases the proliferation of T-lymphocytes. It is useful in a combination regimen to treat colon cancer.

11
Toxicology

I. EMERGENCY TOXICOLOGY

A. The **goals of treatment** of a patient who has been exposed to a toxic substance are (in sequential order):

1. **Control the symptoms,** including
   a. Cardiovascular changes
   b. Loss of respiratory function
   c. Convulsions
   d. Acidosis

2. **Reduce the absorption** of the substance

3. **Administer an antidote** (see Table 11–1)

4. **Enhance the elimination** of the substance

B. Several approaches are available to **reduce the systemic absorption of an ingested toxic substance.**

1. **Chemical adsorption with activated charcoal** can be utilized.
   a. Charcoal binds many, but not all, toxic substances.
   b. One limitation is that charcoal will also bind emetics, antidotes, and dietary substances.

2. **Emesis** can be induced.
   a. **Syrup of ipecac** acts as a local irritant on the gastrointestinal (GI) tract and stimulates the chemoreceptor trigger zone (CTZ) in the CNS to induce vomiting.
      (1) It is sold without a prescription.
      (2) It should be administered as soon as possible, and less than 4 hours after ingestion, to maximize the recovery of the toxic substance.
   b. **Apomorphine** is much less useful as an emetic, because
      (1) Parenteral administration is required.
      (2) Respiratory depression, as with other narcotics, can occur.
   c. Emesis has several **contraindications,** including:
      (1) Ingestion of a **strong acid or alkali**
      (2) Ingestion of a **low viscosity petroleum distillate** (e.g., kerosene), which could be aspirated during emesis
      (3) An **unconscious** patient
   d. The primary **complication** of emesis is **aspiration** of the stomach contents, which can lead to pneumonitis.

3. **Gastric lavage** (pumping the stomach) is also effective.

Table 11-1
Pharmacological Antidotes

Drugs	Antidotes
Acetaminophen	N-Acetylcysteine
Anesthetic-induced malignant hyperthermia	Dantrolene
Anticholinergics	Physostigmine
Arsenic	Dimercaprol or penicillamine
Benzodiazepines	Flumazenil
Carbamates	Atropine
Competitive muscle relaxants	Neostigmine
Cyanide	Nitrite & thiosulfate
	Digoxin immune F_{ab}
Digoxin	Ethanol
Ethylene glycol	Aminocaproic acid
Fibrinolytics	Protamine
Heparin	
	Nitrite
Hydrogen sulfide	Glucagon
Insulin-induced hypoglycemia	Deferoxamine
Iron	Pyridoxine
Isoniazid-induced neuritis	
Lead	$CaNa_2EDTA$, dimercaprol, penicillamine or succimer
Mercury	Dimercaprol or penicillamine
Methanol	Ethanol
Methotrexate	Leucovorin
	Atropine
Muscarine	Methylene blue
Nitrate-induced methemoglobinemia	Naloxone
Opiates	Atropine & pralidoxime
Organophosphates	
	Epinephrine
Penicillin-induced anaphylaxis	Propranolol
Thyroxine	Physostigmine ± lidocaine
Tricyclic antidepressants	Vitamin K
Warfarin	

   a. Lavage should be performed **as soon as possible.**

   b. The **contraindications are the same** as for emesis, except it can be performed in a comatose patient.

   c. **Aspiration of the stomach contents** can also occur with this method.

4. Water can be used to dilute a toxic substance, especially a strong acid or base.

5. Osmotic cathartics will reduce the absorption by enhancing the elimination of a toxic substance in the feces, but this is often ineffective.

C. Elimination of toxic substances from the circulation **can occasionally be hastened.**

   1. The rate of **metabolism** of a toxic substance usually cannot be affected, although the hepatotoxicity of acetaminophen can be reduced by this mechanism.

   a. With an **overdose of acetaminophen,** glutathione will be depleted. This results in the build-up of a reactive intermediate that induces a **delayed hepatotoxicity.**

   b. **Acetylcysteine,** administered shortly after exposure to acetaminophen, will replenish the glutathione, enhance the conjugation of the reactive acetaminophen intermediate, and reduce the hepatotoxicity.

2. The **urinary excretion** of a toxic substance can occasionally be enhanced by:
   a. Osmotic or loop diuretics which will increase urine flow and enhance clearance of a toxic substance by the kidney.
   b. **Changing the pH** of the urine which will enhance the elimination of some toxic substances by ion trapping (converting the substance to the charged form, which cannot be reabsorbed across the nephron wall).
      (1) To be effective, the pK_a of the toxic substance should be **near 7.5** and the V_d must be small.
      (2) **Bicarbonate** enhances the elimination of the **salicylates and phenobarbital** (weak acids).
      (3) **Ammonium chloride** enhances the elimination of **phencyclidine and amphetamines** (weak bases).

3. Hemodialysis or peritoneal **dialysis** can be effective if the toxin:
   a. Is a small molecule and readily crosses membranes
   b. Has a small V_d, so much of the substance is in the serum
   c. Has low protein binding, so much of the substance is in the free form.

4. Hemoperfusion can also be performed.

II. HEAVY METAL TOXICITY AND CHELATORS

A. **Chelators are substances that bind heavy metals.** When heavy metals have been absorbed, chelators are administered for therapeutic purposes. A metal-chelate complex is formed, which is then **excreted.**

   1. **Dimercaprol** (*BAL*) chelates arsenic, mercury, gold, and lead. It must be administered **parenterally.**

   2. **Penicillamine** (*Cuprimine, Depen*) chelates arsenic, mercury, gold, lead, and copper.
      a. It can be administered **orally.**
      b. A penicillin allergy can develop.
      c. Wilson's disease is an indication for use.

   3. **Deferoxamine** (*Desferal*) chelates iron.
      a. It must be administered **parenterally.**
      b. Hemochromatosis is an indication for use.

   4. Edetate calcium disodium (**EDTA**) (*Calcium Disodium Versenate*) binds many heavy metals, but is used primarily to treat lead poisoning.
      a. It must be administered **parenterally.**
      b. **Nephrotoxicity** is a major limitation of this chelator.

B. **Heavy metals form chelates with natural substances in the body.** It is this phenomenon which leads to their toxicity.

   1. **Lead** is handled much like calcium in the body.
      a. **Accumulation** occurs first **in soft tissues** (e.g., kidney), and then **in bone, teeth, and hair.**
      b. Lead can be mobilized from bone by parathyroid hormone.
      c. **Chronic poisoning** from lead is the most common problem, and the symptoms are diverse and non-specific, including:
         (1) **Neurologic effects** (e.g., mental retardation, especially in children)
         (2) **Peripheral neuritis**
         (3) **GI lead colic**
         (4) **Nephropathy**
         (5) **Anemias**
      d. **Treatment** involves the use of chelators.

(1) Both **calcium disodium EDTA** and **dimercaprol** are used initially.
(2) **Sodium EDTA is not used** because it will chelate endogenous calcium and can induce hypocalcemic tetany.
(3) Long-term deleading is performed with **oral penicillamine** or oral succimer (*Chemet*), another lead chelator.

2. **Mercury** forms covalent bonds with sulphur-containing compounds.
  a. **Cell membranes and enzymes** (e.g., cytochrome oxidase) are damaged.
  b. **Acute poisoning** can occur by several routes of exposure.
    (1) Ingestion of mercury induces a **GI syndrome.**
    (2) Inhalation induces a **pneumonitis.**
    (3) **Renal tubular necrosis** occurs with any route of exposure.
  c. **Chronic poisoning** leads to:
    (1) **Neurologic complications,** especially with methylmercury, which is very lipid-soluble.
    (2) **Nephrotoxicity**
  d. **Treatment** of acute mercury poisoning involves the administration of:
    (1) **Fluids**
    (2) **Chelators**
      (a) **Dimercaprol** is used for mercury salt poisoning.
      (b) **Penicillamine** is used for mercury vapor poisoning.
      (c) None are effective for methylmercury poisoning.

3. **Arsenic** binds sulfhydryl groupings leading to enzyme inhibition, or substitutes for phosphate in adenosine triphosphate (ATP).
  a. **Acute** poisoning induces:
    (1) **GI syndromes**
    (2) **Circulatory collapse**
  b. **Chronic** arsenic poisoning leads to **peripheral neuropathies.**
  c. A diagnostic feature is a **garlic odor** on the breath.
  d. **Treatment** of acute arsenic poisoning involves the administration of:
    (1) **Fluids**
    (2) **Vasopressors**
    (3) **Dimercaprol**
  e. **Treatment** of chronic arsenic poisoning involves the administration of **dimercaprol or penicillamine.**

4. **Iron** is very corrosive to the GI tract if taken in high dosages.
  a. **Acute** ingestion induces a **hemorrhagic GI necrosis,** resulting in the development of **shock and metabolic acidosis.**
  b. **Treatment** involves:
    (1) **Lavage with bicarbonate,** which yields ferrous carbonate, a substance that is not absorbed
    (2) **Fluids**
    (3) **Correction of the acidosis**
    (4) **Deferoxamine**

III. OTHER TOXIC SUBSTANCES

A. **Carbon monoxide** induces hypoxia.

1. It acts by:
  a. **Forming carboxyhemoglobin.** The affinity of carbon monoxide for hemoglobin is 200 times greater than the affinity of oxygen for hemoglobin.
  b. **Decreasing the dissociation of oxygen** from oxyhemoglobin.

2. Treatment for carbon monoxide toxicity involves one of the following:
  a. Inhalation of fresh air
  b. Artificial ventilation
  c. 100% oxygen, which shortens the half-life of the carboxyhemoglobin

B. **Cyanide** has a high affinity for ferric (Fe^{3+}) iron.

  1. **Cytochrome oxidases** in mitochondria, which contain Fe^{3+}, are inhibited.
    a. Cellular respiration is decreased.
    b. A cytotoxic hypoxia is induced.

  2. The specific **treatment** for poisoning includes administration of:
    a. A nitrite to induce **methemoglobinemia;** which binds cyanide, drawing it off the cytochrome oxidases
    b. **Thiosulfate,** which converts the cyanide on the methemoglobin to thiocyanate. The thiocyanate is then excreted.

C. **Hydrogen sulfide** also **inhibits cytochrome oxidases. Treatment** involves the administration of **nitrites** to induce **methemoglobinemia,** which binds the sulfide.

D. **Carbon tetrachloride** (a halogenated hydrocarbon) has many toxic effects.

  1. **Acute** poisoning leads to:
    a. **CNS depression** with respiratory depression
    b. **Arrhythmias,** due to the sensitization of the myocardium to catecholamines

  2. **Chronic** poisoning leads to a disruption of cell membranes, resulting in:
    a. **Hepatotoxicity**
    b. **Nephrotoxicity**

E. Dichlorodiphenyltrichloroethane **(DDT) is very lipid soluble.**

  1. It is **concentrated in fat.**
    a. Elimination from the body is extremely slow (1% / day).
    b. It gets into the **food chain,** and biomagnification occurs.

  2. **Acute** toxicity results from the **blockade of potassium permeability changes** in nerve membranes. This can induce tremors and convulsions, although death does not occur in humans.

F. **Paraquat** increases the formation of a **superoxide anion radical** which attacks lipids and produces **pulmonary injury.**

G. **Thalidomide** is a teratogen which **alters organogenesis** (the action of most teratogens), leading to **phocomelia.**

Index of Drugs

*Chapter number & section in text.